Renal Diet For Beginners & Atkins Diet

The ultimate cookbook to Lose Weight, Improve Health and Life, Boost Kidney Functions With Low Sodium and Potassium Recipes

By

Maria Cox

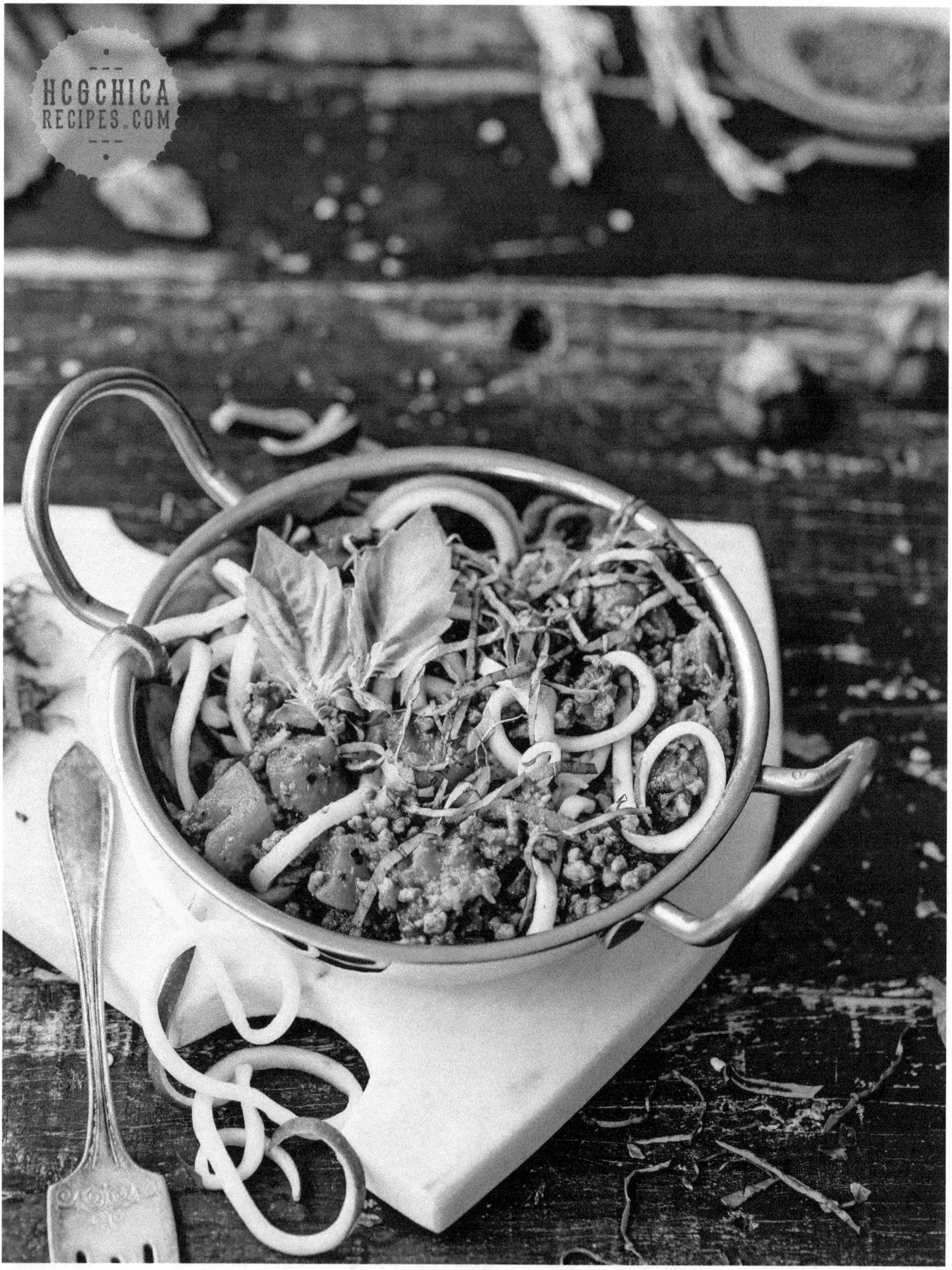
HCGCHICA
RECIPES.COM

TABLE OF CONTENTS

ATKINS DIET FOR BEGINNERS

RENAL DIET COOKBOOK FOR BEGINNERS

Atkins Diet for Beginners

The Complete Beginners Guide With Quick And Tasty Low- Carb, High-Fat Recipes For Busy People To Make at Home

By

Maria Cox

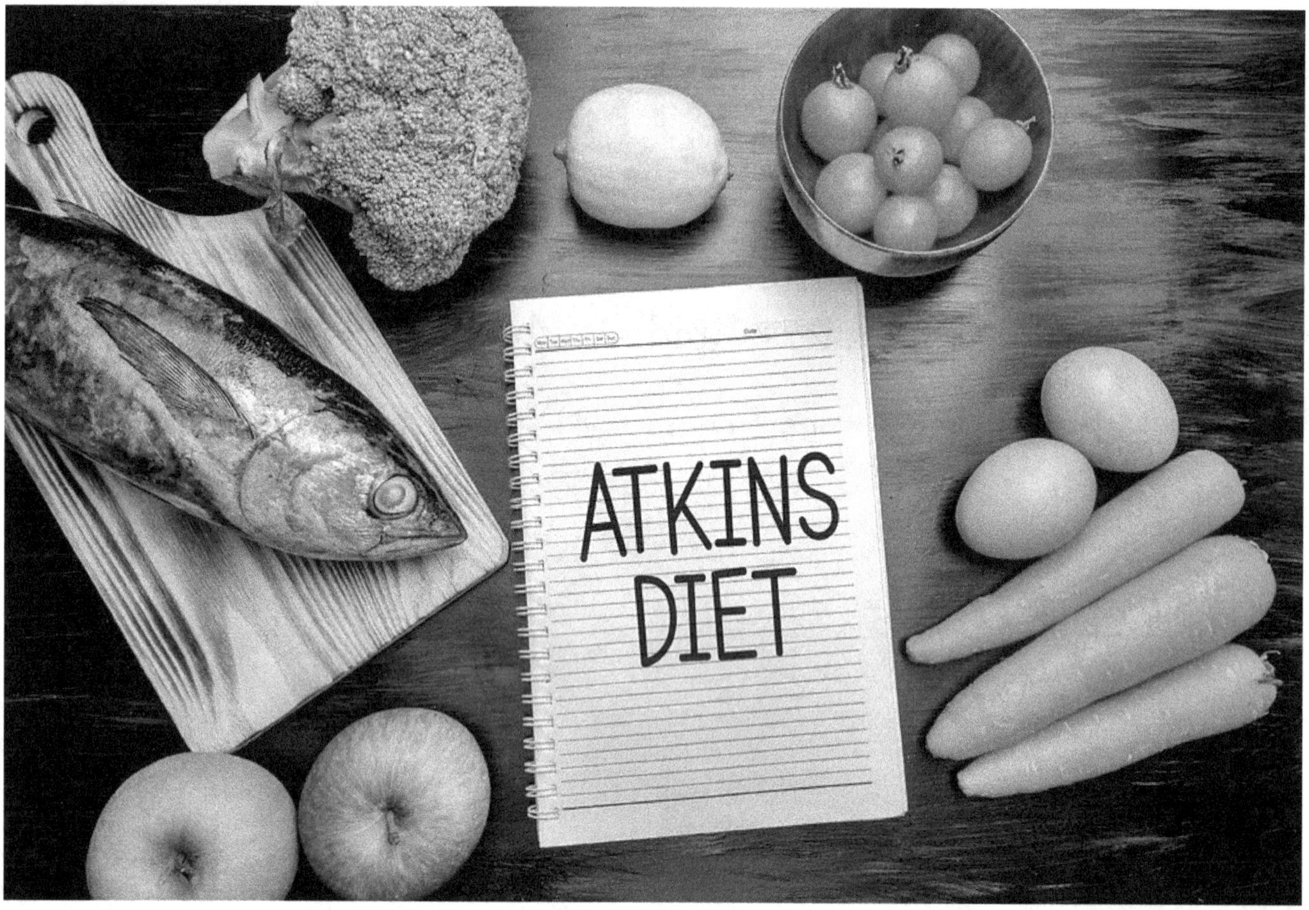
ATKINS
DIET

Introduction

Given the reality that there are well over 1000 reported diets for weight reduction in lay literature, few have gained as much coverage as the Atkins Diet. This high-protein, low-carbohydrate weight-loss diet, which was published in his best-selling novel, The Atkins Diet Revolution, was created by the late Dr. Robert C. Atkins advocated the plan as an easy weight loss diet and a permanent improvement in nutrition. The diet has become increasingly common, enabling people to consume large amounts of meat and high-fat items without taking calorie limits into account. The plan was pointed to by opponents as a high-protein, low-carbohydrate ketogenic, high-fat diet that might be harmful. Without scientific proof, early arguments from both sides were mostly filled by perception and personal perceptions. Eventually, the advent of several clinical studies demonstrated the effectiveness and protection of the Atkins Diet in the research literature. The Atkins diet is a low-carb diet, typically prescribed for weight reduction. A common low carbohydrate eating plan is the Atkins Diet. Although stressing protein and fats, the Atkins Diet excludes carbs (carbohydrates). Proponents of this plan say that, as long as one skip foods rich in calories, he or she will lose weight beside consuming as much fat and protein as one would like.

For weight reduction and maintenance, the Atkins Diet has many stages, beginning with a fairly low carbohydrate eating schedule. In several books, the Atkins Diet, officially named the Atkins Nutritional Method, has been presented in-depth and is credited with initiating the wave of low-carb diets.

About 20 research have demonstrated in the past 12 or so years that low-carb diets without any need for calorie counting are successful for weight reduction and may contribute to numerous health improvements. The diet, primarily because of its high saturated fat content, was initially deemed harmful and demonized by the conventional health authorities. New findings, however, indicate saturated fat is safe. The diet has also been extensively researched and proven to contribute to further weight reduction and better improvements than low-fat diets in blood sugar, 'healthy' HDL cholesterol, triglycerides, and other health markers. Although being rich in fat, on average, it may not increase "bad" LDL cholesterol, but this happens in a subset of people.

The key explanation that low-carb diets are so good for weight reduction is that a decrease in carbohydrates and improved protein consumption contribute to lowered appetite, without needing to worry about it, helping you eat fewer calories. Dr. Robert C. Atkins popularized a high-protein, low-carbohydrate, high-fat weight reduction diet that provides for limitless amounts of beef, eggs and cheese while severely reducing carbs, including candy, flour, noodles, milk, vegetables, and fruits.

Chapter 1: The Atkins Diet

The Atkins diet is based on the notion that insulin development is increased by consuming carbs, which contributes to appetite, eating, and weight gain. The hypothesis is that people experience diminished hunger on the Atkins diet and their bodies use processed fat for energy compared to burning glucose from consumed carbohydrates. It is claimed that consuming fat for energy results in weight loss.

1.1 Why should we choose Atkins diet?

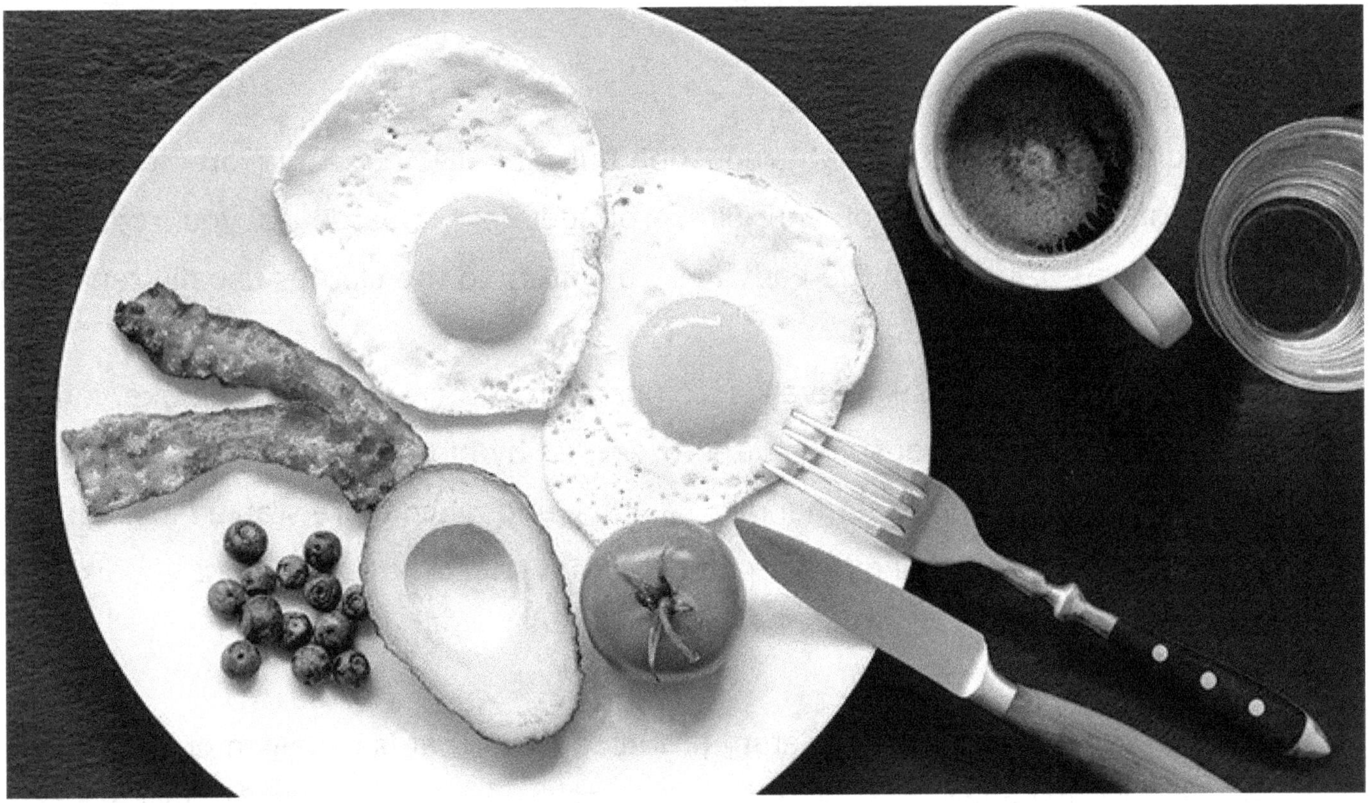

One could opt to stick to the Atkins Diet because:

1. Enjoy the kinds and quantities of food included in the diet.
2. To help you lose weight, you want a diet that reduces those carbohydrates.
3. Want to modify the general eating patterns.
4. Had medical problems that you agree the diet will help change.
5. Like the related products from Atkins Diet, such as cookbooks, bars, and shakes.

If you are starting on Atkins, they will help you during the initial transition period, especially when you have been used to a high carb diet, where you might be craving sugar. Your cravings should fade after a few weeks on Atkins, but even then, low carb snacks will also play a major role by filling the stopgap in meals, so you do not get over hungry.

To help you lose weight and hold it off, the Atkins Diet is meant to modify your dietary patterns. Suppose you choose to reduce weight, maximize your stamina, or help strengthen some health conditions, along with high blood pressure and metabolic disease. In that case, the Atkins Diet often claims it is a safe lifelong approach to food.

Fewer carbs carry major benefits:

Atkins diet contributes to weight reduction but may also have a favorable knock-on impact on other aspects of your life. You get less bloated as you reduce the carbohydrates. Carbs help the body absorb water, so the clothes usually tend to fit better after a week or so.

A sudden increase in insulin levels accompanied by a crash that can make you feel weak, irritable, and exhausted is often triggered by high carb meals. You appear to have more stamina and fewer hunger cravings, and much more stable blood glucose levels. You may have found that the more candy you ingest, the more you like, but that sensation is gone, so it is a lot simpler to stick to Atkins.

Low carb meals filling:

As you consume foods high in dietary protein and fat that is usually more filling, you prefer not to feel hungry on Atkins anyway. The meals and treats you will eat are wonderful and not the typical boring meals that will make you fascinated with food. Plus, because you minimize the carbohydrates you consume, it is often simple to follow Atkins since you do not measure the grams or calories of proteins and fats. Before beginning some weight-loss plan, consult with the primary care doctor professional since it will be even safer.

1.2 How does the Atkins diet works:

One of the well-known low-carb diets is the Atkins diet, and evidence suggests it can benefit. This diet could be the jump-start users need to lose weight if you load your day with refined carbohydrates such as white bread, noodles, and white potatoes and you do not consume enough fruits and vegetables.

When a human practice the Atkins Diet, their body's metabolism changes from consuming sugar, or glucose, as fuel to burning accumulated body fat. Ketosis is considered this switch.

Insulin levels are often down while glucose levels are low, and ketosis happens. In other terms, the body turns to utilize its fat reserves and saturated fats for energy while glucose levels are poor. This will, in turn, help a person lose excess weight and fat.

The glucose levels are low when human eats because their insulin levels have dropped as well. Their glucose levels increase while the individual consumes food, and the body generates more insulin into the bloodstream to help it utilize glucose.

You should avoid the normal go-to items and resume with the Atkins diet page. In food choices, the Atkins 20 plan's initial stage is minimal but based on low carb protein, vegetables, and fats that are not starchy. You add food groups to each stage: first nuts, seeds, berries, then fruits, starchy vegetables, whole grains, and beans. You will select from a greater range of foods and carbohydrates for the Atkins 40 package, but also with little or no starchy foods.

The closest you get to your weight loss target, the more range of foods you are allowed, with Atkins 20. Hopefully, you are trying to adhere to a balanced list and not go back to the old ways.

If you enjoy the wide variety of foods you consume, the Atkins 40 diet may be best for you. Of course, the portion sizes would also need to be held under check, which could be simpler since a low-carb diet can tend to tame appetite.

1.3 Is It good for certain Health conditions?

Shedding pounds will boost your health while you are overweight, and we know the Atkins diet succeeds. Although it is also unknown how long-term health is influenced by the greater amounts of animal fat and protein in the Atkins diet.

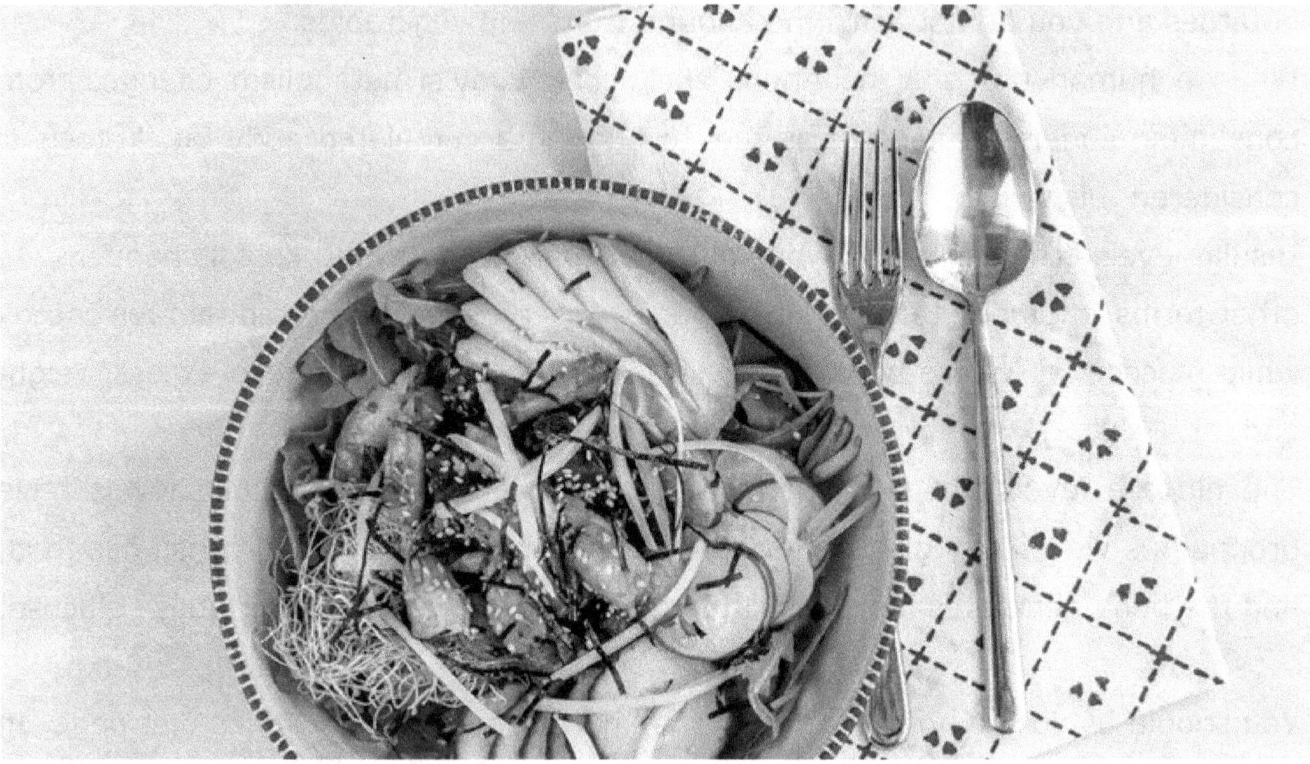

New evidence shows that those who preferred diets high in plant protein and fat on the Atkins diet did better for their health than others who went for the meat fat and protein-rich diet.

This concept is represented by the Atkins 20 and Atkins 40 diets. They rely mostly on consuming fats and protein from heart-healthy options such as olive oil and protein such as soy and lentils.

Before starting this plan, speak to the doctor, whether you have asthma, heart disease, renal disease, or elevated cholesterol, to guarantee that the balance of calories, fat, and protein is good for you.

1.4 Diet details:

For successful fat loss and health, the Atkins Diet's plan primary nutritional emphasis is eating the proper combination of carbs, protein, and fats. The Atkins diet allows one to lose weight by limiting sugar consumption, causing one to burn fat for energy instead of sugar. It often serves, in principle, to reduce cravings for those items. Obesity and associated health conditions like type 2 diabetes and cardiovascular failure are the faults of the traditional high-carbohydrate, low-fat American diet, as per the Atkins Diet. You do not need to skip fatty cuts of meat or cut off extra weight, as per the Atkins Diet. Instead of it controlling carbohydrates, is what is essential. The Atkins Diet proposes that consuming too many carbohydrates contributes to blood glucose imbalances, excess weight and cardiac problems, particularly white flour, sugar, and other processed carbs. The Atkins Diet reduces sugars to the end and recommends consuming more protein and fat. The Atkins Diet states, though, that this is not a high-protein diet.

The Atkins Diet tends to change, like all diet programs. It now promotes more high-fiber vegetables to be consumed, accommodates vegan and vegetarian desires, and tackles health risks that might occur when a low-carb diet is begun.

Carbohydrates:

There is no portion control or calorie counting needed for the Atkins Diet. However, it does require you to watch your carbs. It utilizes a method named net carbs, which is the overall content of an item's carbohydrate minus its fiber content. For instance, there are 2.3 grams of total carbohydrate and 1.3 grams of fiber in a quarter (4 ounces) of raw broccoli, placing its total carbs value at 1 gram.

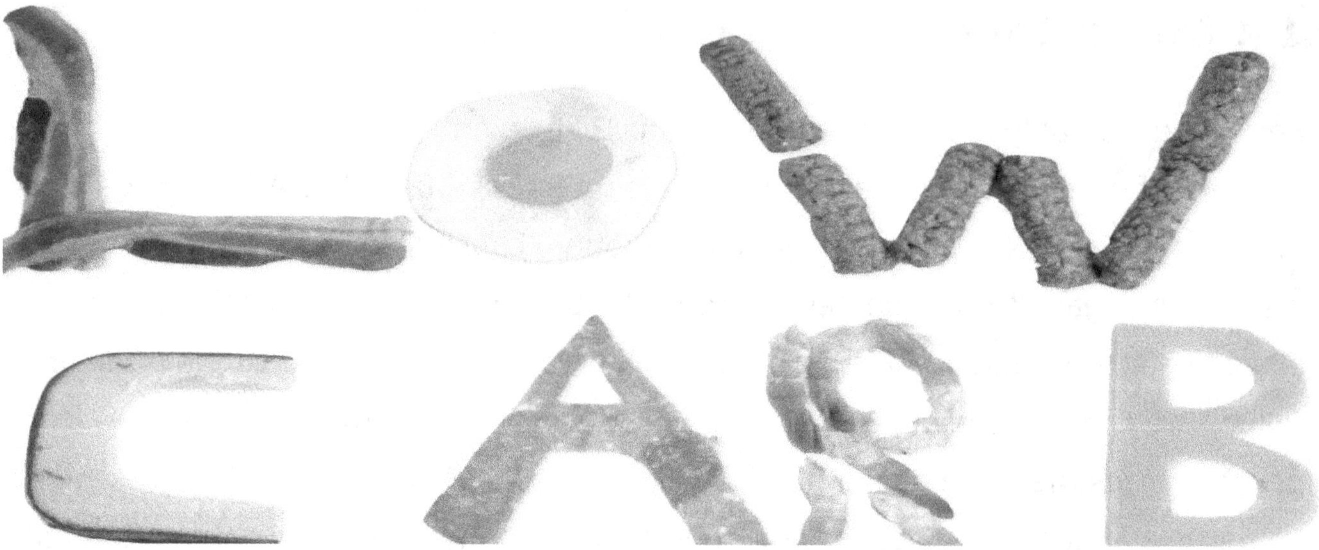

The Atkins Diet claims its carbohydrate solution would burn off the fat reserves in your body, monitor your blood sugar and help you maintain maximum fitness while not keep you feeling hungry or tired. The Atkins Diet also claims that it can help you determine your specific carbohydrate tolerance until you are at your target weight, the number of grams of net carbohydrates you should consume every day without adding or losing weight.

Exercise:

Exercise is not essential for weight reduction; the Atkins Diet says. It agrees, though, that exercising will help you control your weight and have other medical benefits.

1.5 Phases of the Atkins Diet:

The Atkins diet is separated into four distinct stages. If you have a BMI that is healthy? Then it is best to join Atkins' phase 3 or phase 4. The aim is to control your weight in these periods and become even more energetic. Are you obese, or do you want to easily drop weight? Atkins diet recommends beginning with phase 1 (where one can drop weight quickly) or phase 2. (in which one can lose more weight with time). The Atkins Diet's theory is that the body will drive to burn your fat reserves for energy if you count and limit carbohydrates, the natural fuel of the body, thereby encouraging weight loss. The key point is to avoid consuming processed flour and sugar, as with many other fad diets. But carb-dense whole-grain items are on the do not-eat list before one hit the maintenance level unless one attempts to obey the Atkins 20. There are four levels of The Atkins Diet. One may start with either of the initial three steps, depending on the weight loss goals.

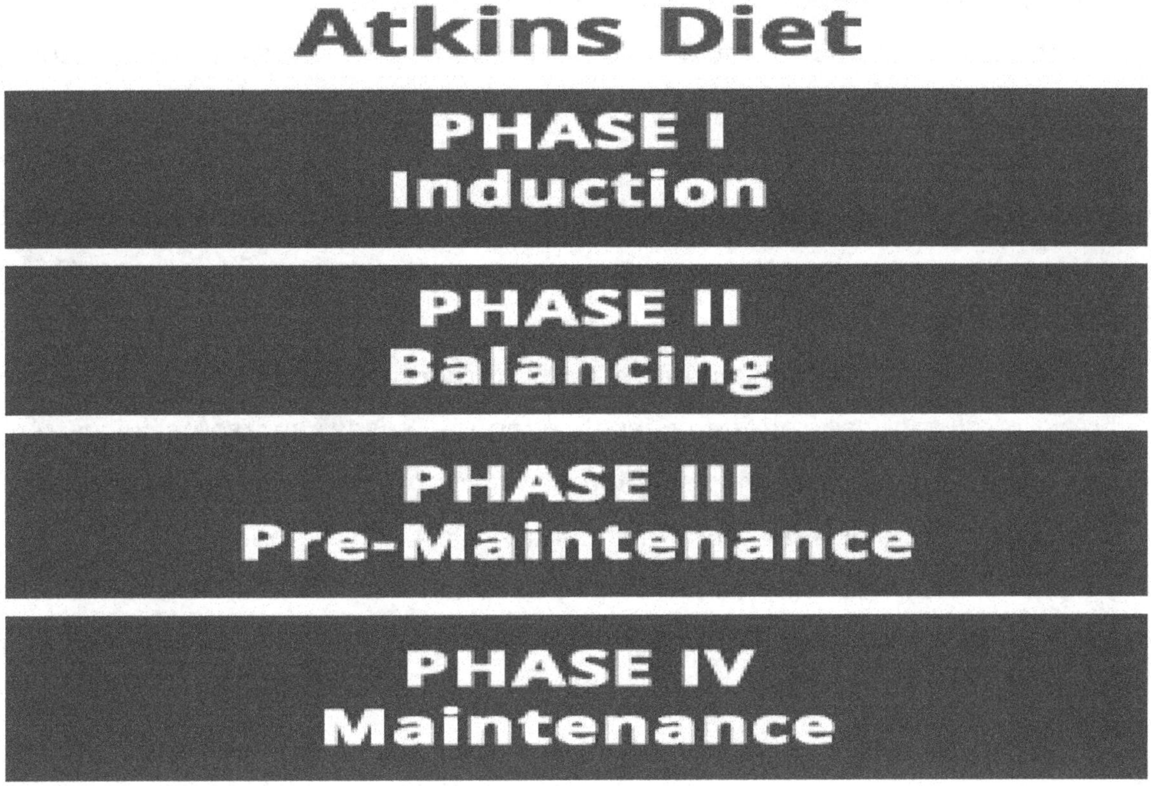

1. **Phase 1: The Induction phase.** Under 20 grams a day of carbohydrate for two weeks. Eat high-protein, high-fat leafy greens such as low-carb carrots. This kick-start the reduction of weight. Users cut out with almost all carbohydrates from the diet in this strict process, consuming just 20 grams of net carbs a day, mostly from vegetables. They get just about 10 percent instead of having 45 to 65 percent of the daily energy from carbs, as prescribed for most diet recommendations. 'Base' vegetables should account for 12 to 15 grams of the daily net carbohydrates, such as asparagus, lettuce, cucumber, celery, green beans, and pepper. Users can consume protein such as fish and shellfish, seafood, beef, eggs, and cheese for every meal. Oils and fats do not need to be regulated, but one cannot include most vegetables, baked products, bread, noodles, wheat, nuts, or alcohol. One must drink eight glasses a day of water. Depending on the weight reduction, users can be in this process for at least two weeks. Because no grain-based foods are tolerated in Phase I, as long as you make sure you stick with gluten-free beverages and gluten-free salad dressing, gluten should not be a concern. The length of induction is up to two weeks.
2. **Phase 2: The Balancing phase:** Add more almonds, low-carb veggies, and limited quantities of fruit back to the diet steadily. In this process, as base vegetables, users continue to eat an average of 12 to 15 grams of carbs. one can probably need to avoid sugar-added items. One should steadily incorporate more veggies and fruit, nuts, and seeds to some nutrient-rich carbohydrates while people begin to lose weight. People continue this process once they are around 4.5 kilograms (10 pounds) from their target weight. One can consume anything they consumed in Phase 1, as in Atkins Phase 2, and incorporate fruit, cottage cheese (make sure you pick up a brand of gluten-free cottage cheese), almonds, seeds, and some juices. Again, no grain-based items are permitted, but one can comfortably eat gluten-free products in this step of the diet if none of the condiments contain gluten.
3. **Phase 3: The Pre-maintenance phase:** Add more calories to the diet while you are close to your target weight before weight reduction slows down. In this process, the variety of foods that one may consume, including starchy vegetables, fruits, and whole grains, will increase steadily. One should add approximately 10 grams of carbohydrates to their diet per week, so they must cut back once the weight reduction stops. If one hits the target weight, they remain in this process. Stage three of the Atkins diet is mainly gluten-free. Oats and brown rice are the only grains tolerated.

But one could get into problems on the gluten front if one also reacts to oats or is just not particular about selecting healthy oatmeal. Furthermore, certain people pursuing Atkins tend to fudge a bit by consuming a grain-based reward at this stage in the diet or getting a little sloppy, and this is when they can learn that they are susceptible to gluten (through unpleasant symptoms).

4. **Phase 4: The Lifetime maintenance phase:**

Here, one can eat as many nutritious carbohydrates without regaining excess weight as the stomach can bear. When you hit your target weight, you step through this process, and so you practice this form of eating for good. Some individuals chose to miss the induction stage and, from the beginning, have lots of vegetables and berries. This approach can also be quite effective.
Others tend to only remain forever in the induction process. It is also recognized as a ketogenic, very low-carb diet (keto). Step 4, meanwhile, is the maintenance phase of the diet, which provides for grain-based products, but the official diet plan recommends only wheat pasta, oatmeal, and brown rice. You should probably miss the wheat pasta to add only oatmeal and brown rice to maintain this gluten-free diet component but make sure to choose better quality gluten-free rice. **These stages, however, are a little complicated but are beneficial for the health. As long as people adhere to these phases and menu plans, they should shed weight and hold it off.**

Chapter 2: The Atkins Plan

A drop of carbohydrates is the pillar of the Atkins Plan. The diet has grown over the years to provide two choices at the moment. The initial step (Phase 1, Induction) for Atkins 20 is 20 g of' Net Carbs' (carbohydrate subtract grams of fiber) per day. The Atkins 40 makes 40 g of net carbohydrates a day at the starting stage. A rise in carbohydrates is allowed by both programs. One method introduces ingredients one at a time while the other improves the portion-size carbohydrate limit when persons reach their weight reduction targets.

The lifestyle, often referred to as the Atkins Dietary Approach, comes with three types today.

1. **Atkins 20 is for individuals who:**

- Wants to shed over 40 pounds (lb.).
- Have a waist diameter of more than 40 inches (men) or 35 inches (women).
- Have pre-diabetes or diabetic type 2.

2. **Atkins 40 is for persons who:**

- Wanting to drop less than 40 lb.
- They are pregnant or nursing and choose to lose weight.
- Need a diet for a broader range of foods.

3. **Atkins 100 is for individuals who:**

- Want to keep their established weight.
- They are pregnant.
- Breastfeeding and attempting to hold their weight in check.

2.1 An Overview of the 3 Atkins Diet Plans:

Both forms of the Atkins diet rely on limiting what is considered net carbs (including those in vegetables) and stressing consuming protein and healthier fat types. Atkins describes net carbs as grams of carbs, excluding grams of fibers. When you start to approach your weight reduction target, pick carbohydrates, and introduce them into your diet. Atkins 20 and Atkins 40 involve different stages, while Atkins 100 is known to be a dietary plan and aims for no more than 100 net carbs per day to be eaten. Your initial 'induction' period in Atkins 20 restricts you to 20 grams (g) of net carbs, while your initial induction phase in Atkins 40 limits you to 40 g of net carbohydrates, offering you a little more versatility in the items that you can consume at the outset (including, for example, choosing fruits and some vegetables), You introduce net carbs back to the diet in 5 g increments (20, 25, 30, and so on) in Atkins 20, while in 10 g increments in Atkins 40, you add net carbs back to your diet, describes Lauren Popeck, RD, of Orlando Health, Florida.

The following chart details the diet guidelines for the first step of Atkins 20 (induction). Keep in mind that on Atkins 40, all these foods are deemed suitable (in small quantities).

a) Atkins 20 Food to eat:

You can eat any of the following foods to help jump-start your weight reduction on the Atkins 20:

- Veggies from the base, such as broccoli, lettuce, bok choy and cucumbers
- Protein, including poultry, eggs, and beef.
- Both seafood, including salmon, char, herring, and flounder.
- Butter and olive oil
- Few cheeses, namely cheddar, goat, Parmesan ham and swiss.
- Avoid: fruits such as pineapples and mangoes; starchy vegetables such as potatoes; and grains, initially at least.

b) Atkins 40 Food to eat:

It would be best if you consume any of the above plus the following foods while you are pursuing the Atkins 40 diet (as long as you hold net carbohydrates below 40 g a day).

- Nuts and seeds.
- Legumes (beans)
- Berries
- Starchy plants such as potatoes, carrots, and beets
- Whole grains such as rye, whole-grain rice, and spaghetti of whole wheat
- Avoid fruits such as mangoes and pineapples; starchy vegetables such as starchy grains and potatoes, initially at least.

c) Atkins 100 Food:

As long as you do not surpass 100 g of net carbohydrates a day, Atkins 100 supporters will consume nearly all foods. If you are consuming sugar or processed carbohydrates, carbs will add up easily, so it is better to restrict or stop them. There are no foods on the Atkins 100 that are deemed off limits. Even so, still on Atkins 100, you should expect to hold your carbohydrate consumption below 50 grams a day, but you may need to keep limited amounts of carbohydrate-rich items in order to sustain the target.

Be sure you have in your diet a selection of various vegetables. There are four stages of the conventional Atkins diet, called Atkins 20. You should expect to cut down on your consumption of carbohydrates at each point, but the first, called induction, is the most restricting stage. In later levels, or whether you prefer Atkins 40 or Atkins 100, the consumption of carbohydrates would be better, but much smaller than the USDA's prescribed intake.

Chapter 3: What's In The Menu:

3.1 Preferable Foods:

- Foundational vegetables
- Shellfish and Fish
- Poultry
- Eggs, cream, and cheese
- Oils and fats
- Meat

3.2 Non-preferable Foods:

- Starchy vegetables
- Alcoholic beverages
- Most processed foods
- Seeds and nuts
- Sugary beverages
- Cereals
- Sweet treats and Junk foods
- Fruits and fruit juices
- Condiments, salad dressing and sauces
- Sweetened yogurt
- Grain and grain products
- Lentils and beans
- Crackers and chips

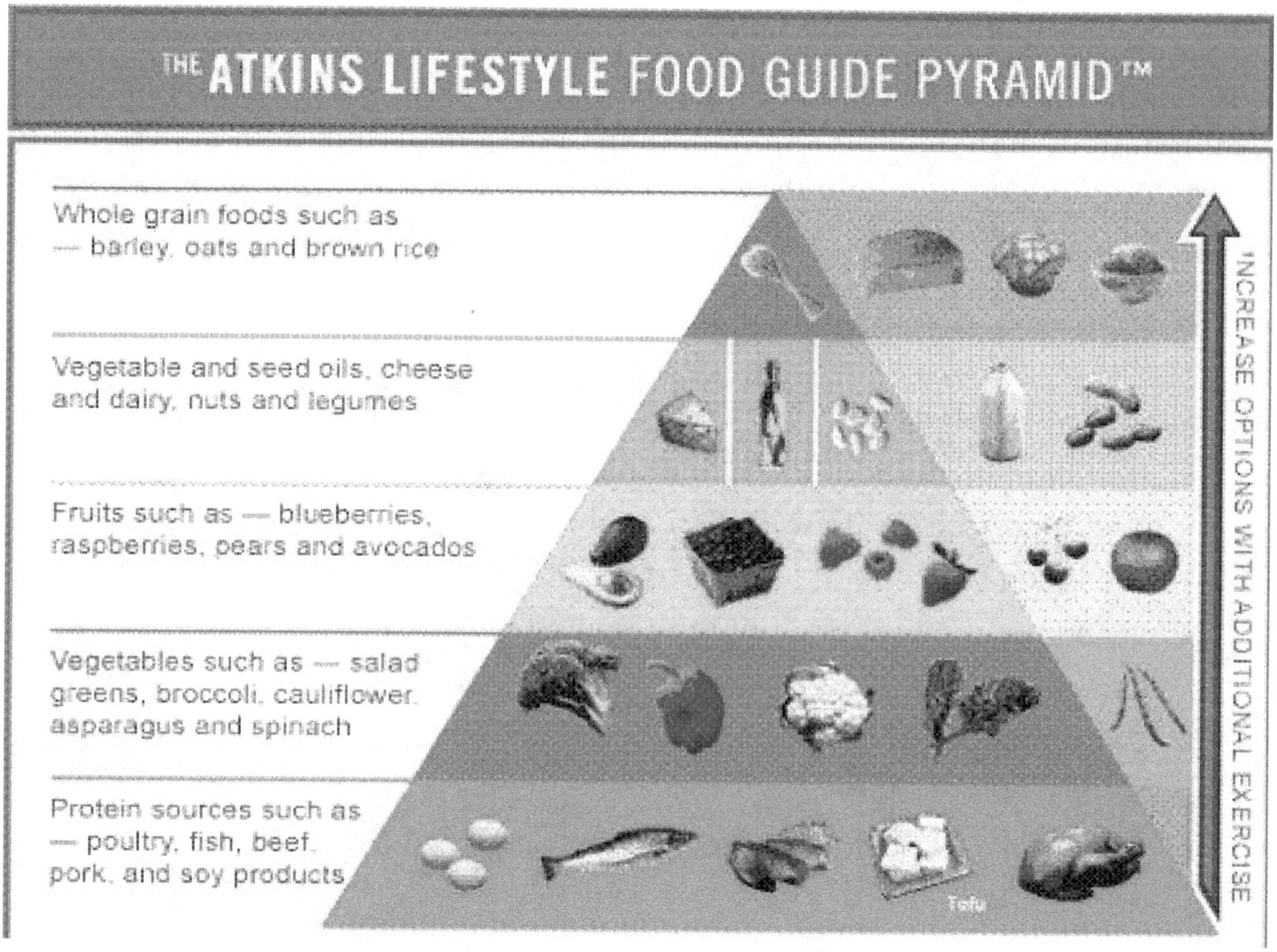
THE ATKINS LIFESTYLE FOOD GUIDE PYRAMID™
Whole grain foods such as — barley, oats and brown rice
Vegetable and seed oils, cheese and dairy, nuts and legumes
Fruits such as — blueberries, raspberries, pears and avocados
Vegetables such as — salad greens, broccoli, cauliflower, asparagus and spinach
Protein sources such as — poultry, fish, beef, pork, and soy products
Tofu
INCREASE OPTIONS WITH ADDITIONAL EXERCISE

1. Preferable Foods:

An easy guide to Atkins 20, the Initial step is this "Acceptable Low Carb Foods List." By growing your
daily net carb consumption to an average of 20g a day, you can kick start induction during this process.

Among these, 12-15 grams must be in the form of foundational vegetables. Enjoy some of the meats, proteins, balanced fats, seeds and nuts, and most cheeses from collecting suitable low carb base vegetables below.
On these balanced ingredients, you can center your diet.

- **Seeds and nuts:** Walnuts, almonds, macadamia nuts, seeds of sunflower etc.
- **Foundational Vegetables**: Cauliflower, broccoli, cabbage, cucumber, brussels sprouts, kale, spinach, asparagus, bok choy, zucchini, olives, eggplant, mushrooms, cucumber, avocado, peppers, tomatoes, onions, lettuce, other leafy greens, etc. These are the lowest containing carbs in net carbohydrates and can be appreciated at all degrees of carb restriction. However, you will need to restrict your portions to certain kinds, such as bell peppers and Brussels sprouts, if you adopt a keto diet (< 20 grams of carbohydrates per day). In the Atkins diet, most carbs come from simple low-carb vegetables such as cabbage, lettuce, asparagus, broccoli, and others. It is important to know the number of carbohydrates in the vegetables that you consume. People at Atkins can aim and eat lettuce, cucumber, mushrooms, zucchini, broccoli, and 12-15 grams of net carbs each day.
- **Shellfish and Fish**: Fish is high in protein and good fats and is an outstanding source of vitamins D and B2, minerals and calcium such as iron and potassium. While all fish are Phase 1 acceptable low carb foods and do not have net carbs, Atkins suggest sticking to the styles mentioned here a few days a week for a 4-6 ounce serving., Because of the large levels of omega-3 fatty acids, fatty fish such as trout, salmon, sardines, mackerel, or herring are fine and may also provide health benefits. Everyone on Atkins is urged to eat a 4–6-ounce portion of seafood. Because of the calorie count, breaded fish is off-limits. However, some fish and shellfish, such as trout, tuna, halibut, cod, or flounder, are preferred. Appropriate foods contain shellfish such as shrimp, lobster, and

clams. Oysters and mussels are all right at this point, but as they are higher in carbohydrates, it is recommended that you limit the intake to four ounces or less.

- **Poultry:** Butter, cheese, milk, full-fat yogurt, full-fat dairy goods are preferable. Atkins recommends that between three meals, you divide the protein consumption and get it from various sources. Fowl is acceptable, like pigeon, turkey, duck, pheasant, and goose. 4–6 ounces are a recommended serving. Remember that cheese produces around 1 gram per ounce of carbohydrate, and Atkins suggests that you eat no more than 3-4 ounces of cheese a day. An ounce is around the size of a 1-inch cube or a slice of American cheese individually packed.
- **Meat:**

A component of the Atkins diet may be beef, pork, lamb, eggs, bacon, and others. Acceptable meat forms include beef, pork, lamb, veal, and venison, and Atkins consumers are urged to serve meat in the correct serving size (4-6 ounces). You ought to be vigilant of some meat forms on the Atkins plan, including pork, sausage, and other cooked meats. These items can include added sugar since sugar is used to cure them. Atkins consumers are also advised to avoid meat containing nitrates and cold meat cuts.

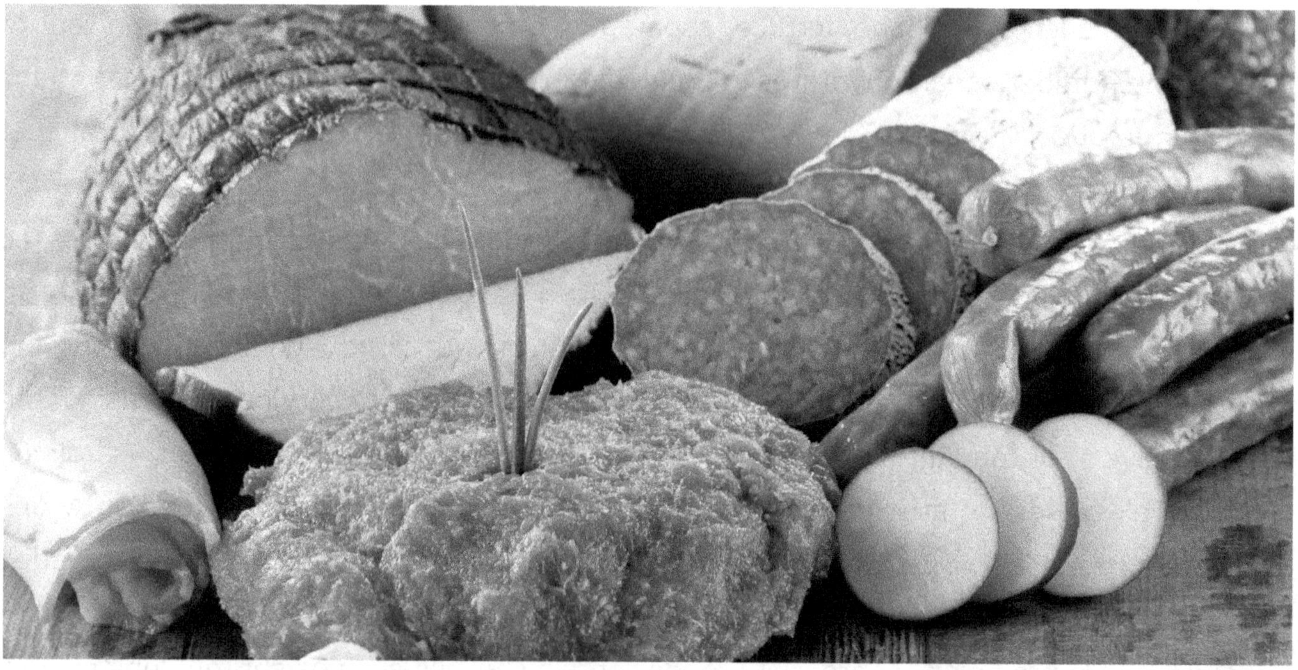

- **Eggs, Cheese and Cream:**

Eggs on Atkins are a preferred protein source, e.g., The healthiest eggs are enriched or pastured with omega 3. There are certain carbs in cheese, but it is recommended for anyone on the plan to eat no more than 3 ounces a day. Any other dairy items may be eaten, such as cream and sour cream, but goat's milk, cottage cheese, yogurt and ricotta are not suggested.

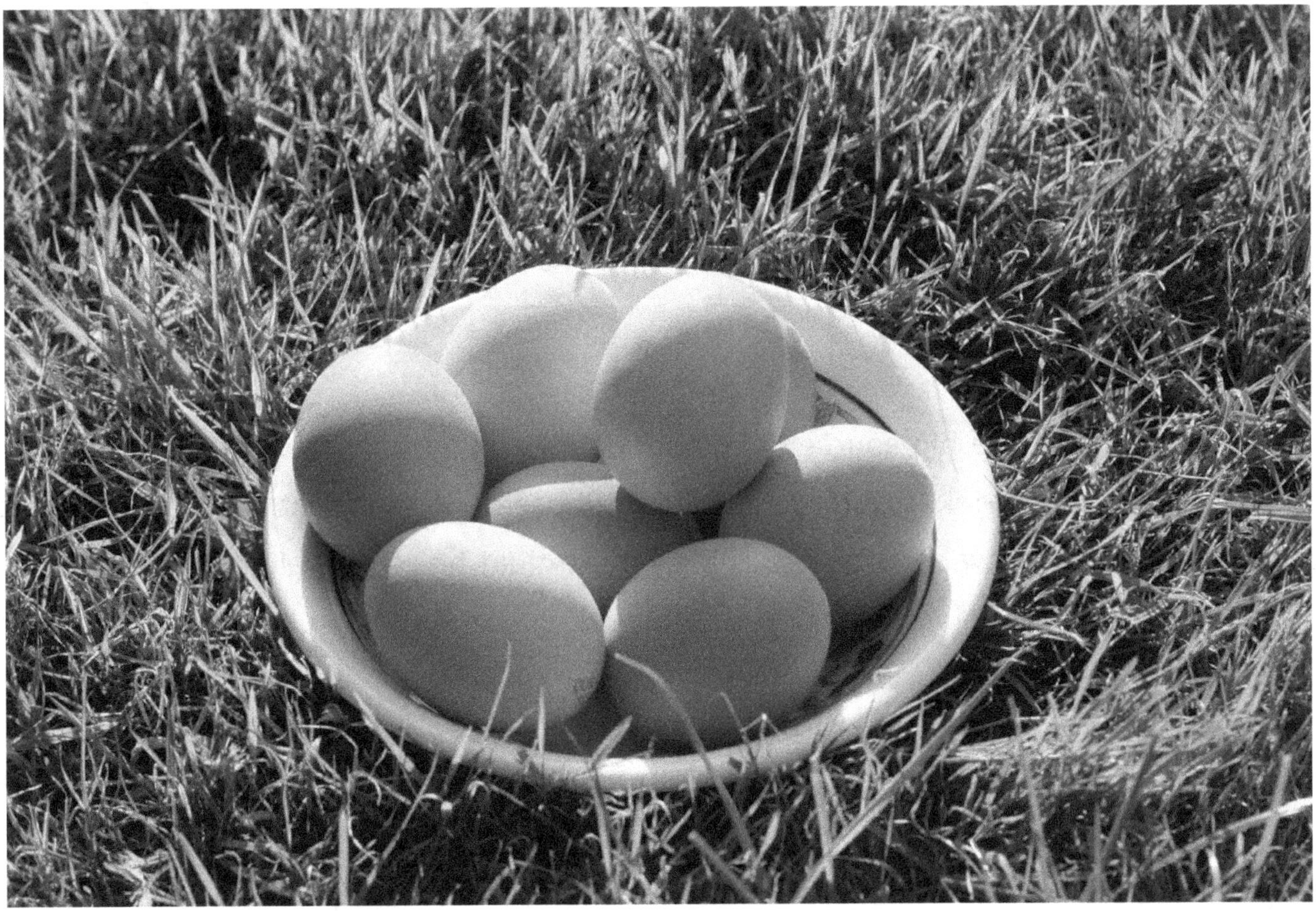

- **Oils and fats:**

A significant aspect of Atkins is to consume a healthy quantity of fat. There are no sugars, but keep in mind that the maximum consumption indicated for added fats is 2-4 teaspoons a day. When cooking, do not encourage any oils to exceed extremely high temperatures and use olive oil to sauté. To dress cooked veggies or lettuce, use walnut or sesame oil, but not for frying. Coconut oil, extra virgin oil, avocados and avocado oil may be part of the diet Atkins. You can lose weight as long as you center your meals on a source of fatty protein with vegetables or nuts and other healthier fats. It is so simple. While there is a common belief that people consume large quantities of butter and other saturated fat on Atkins, this is not accurate. Followers of Atkins are recommended to retain 2-4 teaspoons a day of their added fat consumption. Mayonnaise, butter, olive oil, walnut or sesame oil are suitable fats.

- **Beverages:**

Since they are also a big source of secret sugars and carbohydrates, pay particular attention to your drinks. During Atkins 20, Phase 1, it is essential to consume at least 64 ounces of water a day. Drinking more fluid helps in weight control and is essential for maintaining health. Here are several beverages on the Atkins diet that are suitable.

1. **Water:** As always, the go-to beverage should be water. Keep making IT your drink of choice, as well as flavored or sparkling water, but be sure to read the list of ingredients to search for added sugars.
2. **Coffee**: Several tests indicate that coffee is strong and very high in antioxidants but is healthy. For weight reduction, black or with minimal quantities of milk or cream is optimal. Be sure to add loads of milk or cream, particularly if you often drink coffee during the day, even if you are not hungry. But feel free to use full-fat cream if you are starving. Or try coconut oil and butter called as "Bulletproof coffee".
3. **Green tea**: A very healthy beverage. In limited doses, alcohol is good as well. Stick to dry wines without added sugar and skip beer-like high-carb beverages.

In the Atkins plan, you must limit certain foods:

2. Non-Preferable Foods:

It is essential to select foods rich in nutrients but low in carbohydrates while adopting a low-carb Atkins diet. Few foods should be minimized, and others should be entirely avoided. In part, your decisions rely on your carbohydrate tolerance. Focus on consuming a selection of nutritious foods in the meantime.

- **Grains and Grain Products:**

A large variety of food items made from grains are used in the typical American diet. If you are in the initial step of Atkins 20, you must not eat certain items. Such products include bread, cereal, pasta muffins, bagels, and other baked goods. You are not going to eat carbohydrates like corn, wheat, or barley, too. Bread is a staple food in many countries. It appears in many types, such as loaves, bagels, wraps, and flatbreads, like tortillas. All of these are, however, high in carbohydrates. This is relevant for types of whole grain as well as those produced from processed wheat. While carbohydrate counts differ depending on the portion sizes and ingredients for common bread, here are all the average counts:

- ✓ **Whole-wheat bread (1 slice):** 17 grams of carbohydrates, 2 of them are fiber.
- ✓ **White bread (1 slice):** 14 grams of carbohydrates, 1 of them is fiber.
- ✓ **Bagel (3-inch):** 29 grams of carbohydrates, 1 of them is fiber.
- ✓ **Flour tortilla (10-inch):** 36 grams of carbohydrates, 2 of them are fiber.

Eating a toast, burrito, or bagel could bring you close to or over your daily limit, based on your carb tolerance. Make your low-carb loaves at home if you do want to enjoy the bread. Many grains are often rich in carbohydrates, like rice, wheat, and oats, and should be limited or eliminated on a low-carb diet like the Atkins diet.

Pasta is a staple that is versatile and cheap but very rich in carbohydrates. There are 43 grams of carbs in one cup (250 grams) of cooked pasta, about 3 of them are fiber. At 37 grams of carbohydrates, including 6 grams of fiber, the same quantity of whole-wheat pasta is just a marginally better choice. Eating spaghetti or other pasta forms is not a safe option on a low-carb diet because you eat a really limited amount, which for most people is not possible. Start making shirataki noodles or spiralized vegetables instead if you are wanting pasta but do not want to go off the carb limit. You will learn to use limited grains in your diet while you make progress on Atkins. You are encouraged to use whole grains, which are rich in fiber.

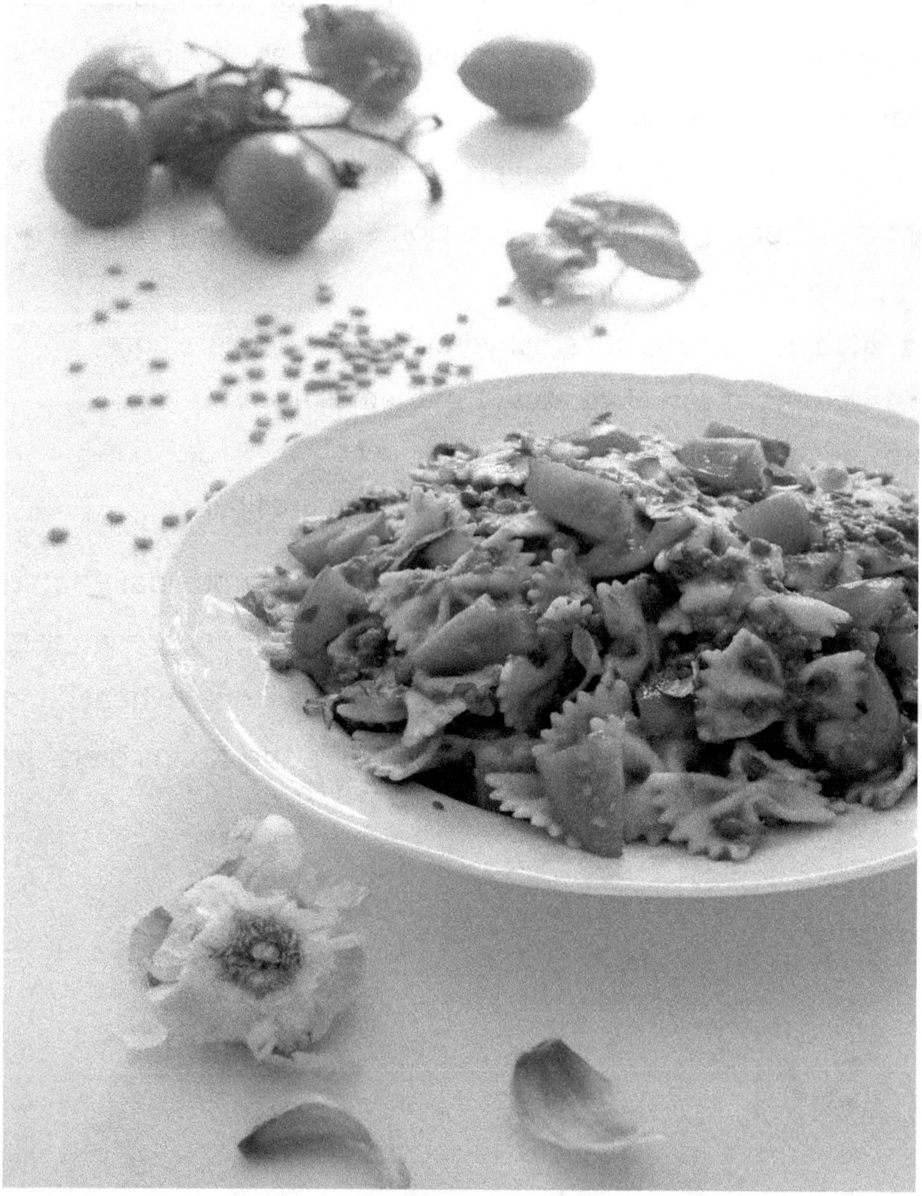

- **Cereal:**

It is well established that several carbohydrates are included in sugary breakfast cereals. You can be shocked, though, by the carb counts of balanced cereals. For example, 32 grams of carbs are provided in 1 cup (90 grams) of cooked, normal, or instant oatmeal, with only four fibers. Steel-cut oats are less refined and are generally considered better than other forms of oatmeal. However, 29 grams of carbs are present in a mere 1/2 cup (45 grams) of cooked steel-cut oats, including 5 grams of fiber. Whole-grain cereals are also more likely to pack even more. A 1/2 cup (61 grams) of granola comprises 37 grams of carbohydrate and 7 grams of fiber, whereas a massive 46 grams of carbohydrate and 5 grams of fiber is filled in the same quantity of grape nuts. A bowl of cereal might easily bring you over your total carb cap, based on your personal carb goal, before milk is added.

- **Fruit and Fruit Juice:**

Higher consumption of and vegetables and fruits has consistently been correlated with a reduced risk of heart failure and cancer. Many vegetables, though, are rich in carbohydrates, which may not be acceptable for low-carb diets, such as the Atkins diet. One small piece or 1 cup (120 grams) is a typical serving of fruit. For instance, a small apple produces 21 grams of carbohydrates, 4 of which come from fiber. It is probably a good idea to eliminate certain fruits on a very low-carb diet, particularly dried fruits, and sweet fruits, with a high carb count.

- ✓ **Mango sliced (1 cup / 165 grams):** 28 grams of carbohydrates, 3 of them are fiber.
- ✓ **Raisins (1 ounce / 28 grams):** 22 grams of carbohydrates, 1 of them is fiber.
- ✓ **Dates (2 large):** 36 grams of carbohydrates, 4 of them are fiber.
- ✓ **Banana (1 medium):** 27 grams of carbohydrates, 3 of them are fiber.

Berries are higher in fiber and lower in sugar than other fruits. Therefore, also on very-low-carb diets, small amounts can be enjoyed, about 1/2 cup (50 grams). In a low-carb diet, the juice is one of the worse drinks you might consume. While it contains certain nutrition, fruit juice is quite rich in fast-digesting carbohydrates, triggering a sudden rise in your blood sugar. E.g., apple juice containing 12 ounces (355 ml) holds 48 grams of carbs. This is also better than a drink holding 39 grams. For a 12-ounce (355-ml) serving, grape juice contains a whopping 60 grams of carbohydrates. While vegetable juice does not produce quite as many carbs as its fruit equivalents, there are still 16 grams of carbs in a 12-ounce (355-ml) serving, just 2 of which come from fiber.

What is more, the juice is another source of liquid carbs that might not be absorbed in the same manner as for solid carbs through your brain's appetite center. Later in the day, consuming juice will result in increased appetite and food consumption. Although there are many essential vitamins in fruit and fruit juice, these fruits and drinks often provide sugars and glucose, making them rich in carbohydrates. In the late stages of Atkins, you may add certain low-carb fruits to the diet; you should fully prevent them in the first phase of Atkins 20.

- **Starchy vegetables:**

Many diets allow an unrestricted consumption of vegetables that are low in starch. Most vegetables are very rich in fiber, which may promote weight loss and regulation of blood sugar. Some high-starch vegetables produce more digestible carb than fiber, but these vegetables on a low-carb diet should be restricted. What is more, if you are adopting a low-carb diet, skipping these starchy vegetables entirely is the safest choice:

- ✓ **Corn (1 cup / 175 grams):** 41 grams of carbohydrates, 5 of them are fiber.
- ✓ **Sweet potato/ 1 medium yam:** 24 grams of carbohydrates, 4 of them are fiber.
- ✓ **Potato (1 medium):** 37 grams of carbohydrates, 4 of them are fiber.
- ✓ **1 cup / 150 grams cooked beets:** 16 grams of carbohydrates, 4 of them are fiber.

Notably, on a low-carb diet, you can enjoy some low-carb vegetables.

- **Beans and Lentils:**

A good source of nutrients and protein is lentils, beans, chickpeas (for example, kidney beans, split peas, or garbanzo beans). However, since these items are often a good source of carbohydrates, most phases of Atkins 20 can inhibit them. Beans and legumes are healthy food. They may have several health advantages, including a lowered risk of inflammation and heart attack. While rich in fiber, they produce a decent quantity of carbs as well. You could be allowed to use minor quantities on a low-carb diet based on personal tolerance. Here are the carb counts for 1 cup (160–200 grams) of legumes and cooked beans:

- ✓ **Peas:** 25 grams of carbohydrates, 9 of them are fiber
- ✓ **Lentils:** 40 grams of carbohydrates, 16 of them are fiber
- ✓ **Pinto beans:** 45 grams of carbohydrates, 15 of them are fiber.
- ✓ **Black beans:** 41 grams of carbohydrates, 15 of them are fiber.
- ✓ **Chickpeas:** 45 grams of carbohydrates, 12 of them are fiber
- ✓ **Pinto beans:** 45 grams of carbohydrates, 15 of them are fiber.

- **Alcoholic Beverages:**

Alcohol on a low-carb diet can be enjoyed in moderation. Currently, dry wine contains very little carbohydrates, and hard liquor has zero. Alcohol is moderately heavy in carbohydrates, though. On average, a 12-ounce (356-ml) can of beer contains 13 grams of carbohydrates. There are also 6 grams of carbs in per can of light beer.

What is more, studies indicate that liquid carbs appear to facilitate weight gain more than solid food carbs. That is because liquid carbohydrates are not as filling as solid food, and the hunger does not appear to reduce almost as much. In the first step of Atkins 20, you will eliminate alcoholic drinks. You will start to appreciate these drinks in moderation and with caution from phase 2 onwards. Simple liquors seem to contain fewer sugars, but with sugar, mixers tend to be produced.

- **Sugary Beverages**

You are already well informed that things rich in sugar, including sweets, candy, and cookies, are off-limits on a low-carb diet. You do not realize that normal sugar contains as many carbs as white sugar. Currently, when weighed in tablespoons, many of them are even richer in carbohydrates.

Here are the carbohydrate counts for one tablespoon of various types of sugar:

- ✓ **Maple syrup:** 13 grams of carbohydrates
- ✓ **White sugar:** 12.6 grams of carbohydrates
- ✓ **Agave nectar:** 16 grams of carbohydrates
- ✓ **Honey:** 17 grams of carbohydrate

What is worse, little, or no nutritional benefit is given by these sweeteners. When carb consumption is minimal, selecting safe, high-fiber carb sources is particularly important. Choose a balanced sweetener instead of sweeteners of foods or drinks without consuming carbohydrates. Any flavored non-alcoholic drinks are made of sugar or chemical sweeteners. Sugary drinks are usually off-limits. Also, drinks produced with artificial sweeteners (sucralose, stevia, or saccharine) are tolerated. It is proposed that followers of Atkins restrict ingestion to the average of three packets a day.

- **Seeds and nuts:**

Another healthy source of fat and protein is nuts and beans, but they also raise carbohydrate consumption. In general, on the induction level of Atkins, they are not advised. However, you will swap three grams of net carbohydrates from vegetables for three grams of nuts or seeds if you have chosen to remain longer than two weeks in this phase.

- **Condiments, sauces, and Salad Dressing:**

On a low-carb diet, a large range of salads may be appreciated daily. Commercial dressings, however, always end up adding more carbs than you would think, particularly low-fat and fat-free types. Two tablespoons (30 ml) of fat-free French dressing, for example, includes 10 grams of carbohydrates. There are 11 grams of carbohydrates in an equal portion of fat-free ranch dressing. More than two tablespoons (30 ml), especially on a broad entrée salad, are widely used by several people. Dress the salad with a creamy, full-fat dressing to minimize the carbohydrates. It is better possible to utilize a splash of vinegar and olive oil, which can support weight control and is related to improved heart health. While several sauces and salad dressings are made from fat, added sugars are often used in most. Ketchup and barbecue sauce, for instance, are often rich in sugar. Salad dressings could also be a source of added sugar. Typically, these items are off-limits unless there is no natural or artificial sugar in them.

- **Sweetened yogurt:**

Yogurt is a versatile and nutritious food. While plain yogurt is comparatively low in carbohydrates, fruit-flavored, sweetened low-fat or non-fat yogurt is also consumed by several individuals. Yogurt that is sweetened also includes as many calories as a dessert. Up to 47 grams of carbohydrate can contain one cup (245 grams) of non-fat sweetened fruit yogurt, much greater than a comparable serving of ice cream. Choosing a 1/2 cup (123 grams) of regular Greek yogurt, though, topped with 1/2 cup (50 grams) of blackberries or raspberries, can keep under 10 grams of digestible carbohydrates.

- **Crackers and chips:**

The famous snack foods are chips and crackers, but their carbohydrates will easily add up. There are 18 grams of carbohydrates in one ounce (28 grams) of tortilla chips, about 1 of which is fiber. This probably 10-15 average-sized chips. Based on processing, crackers differ in carb quality. However, even whole-wheat crackers produce around 19 grams of carbohydrates per 1 ounce (28 grams), plus 3 grams of fiber. Processed snack items are usually eaten within a limited amount of time in significant amounts, so especially if you are on a carb-restricted diet, it is better to avoid them.

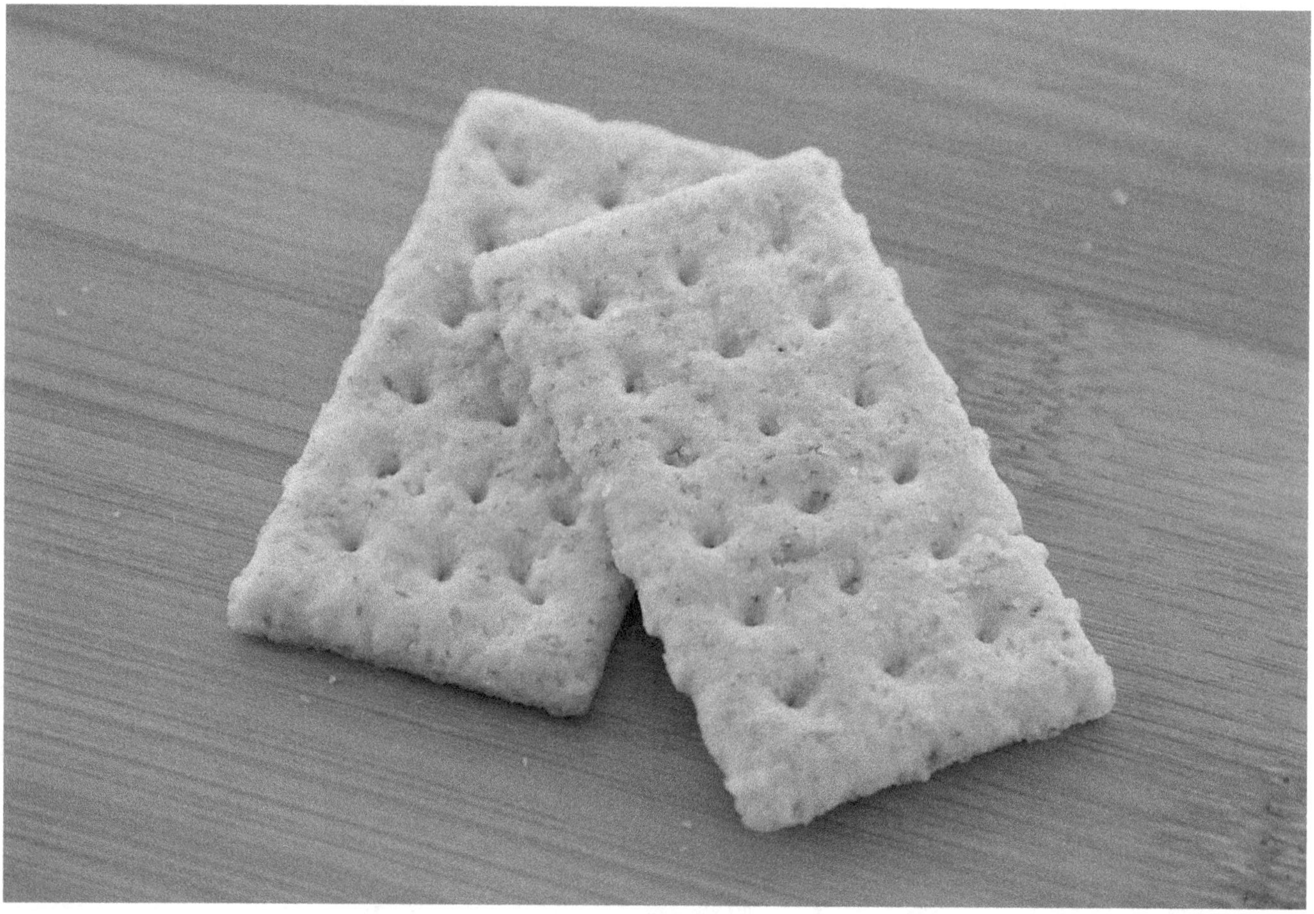

3.3 Food you may eat:

In the Atkins diet, there are many tasty items that you should consume. This involves things such as heavy cream, bacon, dark chocolate, and cheese. Because of the high-calorie content and high fat, most of them are commonly called fattening.

- ✓ **Unrefined grains:** Brown rice, quinoa, oats, and many others.
- ✓ **Tubers:** Sweet potatoes, potatoes, and some others.
- ✓ **Legumes:** Lentils, pinto beans, black beans etc. (if you can bear them).
- ✓ What is more if you want you can have the following in moderation:
- ✓ **Dark chocolate: choose organic products of at least 70% cocoa. Dark chocolate is rich in antioxidants, and if you consume it in moderation, it will have health benefits. However, if you eat too much, be careful that dark chocolate and drugs can inhibit your development.**
- ✓ **Wine: Select dry wines that do not contain artificial sugar or carbohydrates.**

Your liver, though, improves the usage of fat as an energy source while you are on a low-carb diet and suppresses your appetite, decreasing the chance of overeating and weight gain.

3.4 A typical day's menu on the Atkins Diet:

Here is a preview of what you might consume on a normal Atkins Diet day:

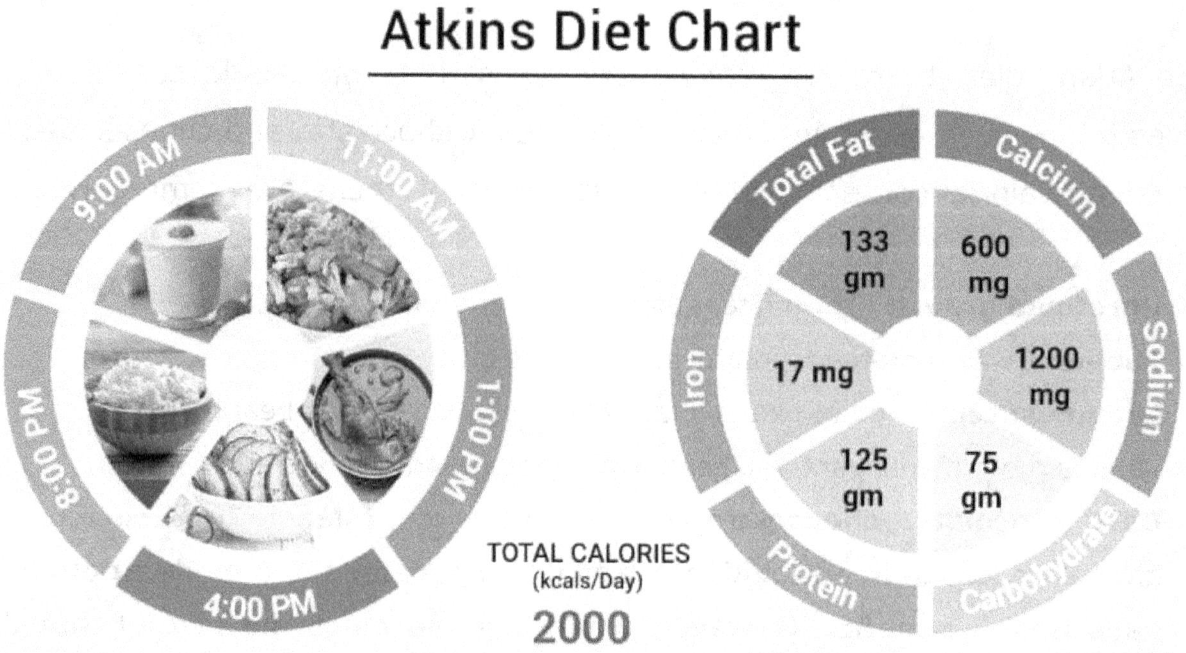

- **For breakfast.** Scrambled eggs sautéed with cheddar cheese and onions. Tea, coffee, water, herbal tea, and diet soda are suitable beverages.
- **Lunch.** Chef's salad with chicken, avocado dressing, and bacon, along with an acceptable beer.
- **Dinner.** Cherry tomatoes and cucumbers with baked salmon steak, arugula salad and asparagus, along with an allowable beer.
- **Snacks.** Usually, you can get two snacks a day. An Atkins Diet product, such as a granola bar or chocolate shake, or a basic snack such as cheddar cheese and celery are acceptable.

3.5 A typical Week's menu on the Atkins diet:

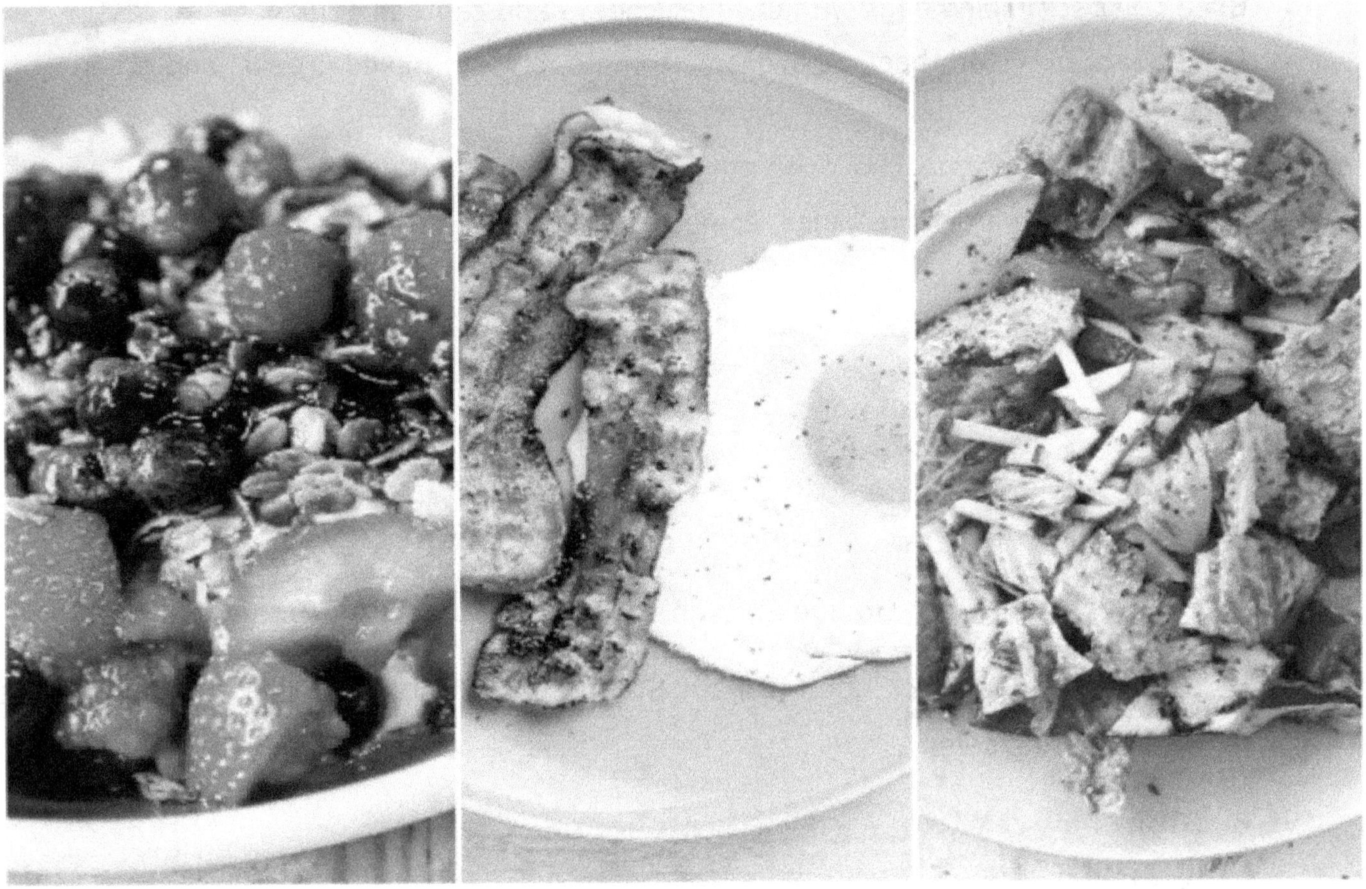

Here's what a week of eating could look like on the Atkins 20 diet.

Day 1

- **Breakfast** Spinach and cheese omelet with salsa and avocado.
- **Lunch** Stir fried chicken roast.
- **Snack** mozzarella string cheese.
- **Dinner** Broccoli and chicken Alfredo with a salad.

Day 2

- **Breakfast** scrambled eggs with cheddar cheese and sautéed onions.
- **Lunch** taco bowl with beef, ½ avocado, tomato, onions, mixed greens, and green peppers
- **Snacks** Atkins Caramel chocolate nut roll Bar: Muffin made within a minute.
- **Dinner** fish with artichoke sauce, spinach, and cauliflower salad.

Day 3

- **Breakfast** Tomato, spinach, avocado and Monterey jack stacks.
- **Lunch** Atkins Frozen Orange Chicken.
- **Snacks** Atkins Milk Choco Delight Shake; 2 tablespoons (tbsp) cream cheese with 2 stalks celery.
- **Dinner** Stuffed Pork Chops with Fennel Gratinata, Fonduta and a broccoli.

Day 4

- **Breakfast** red bell pepper stuffed with spinach and eggs.
- **Lunch** Atkins Chocolate Peanut Butter Bar
- **Snacks** Atkins French Vanilla Shake; 1cup sliced cucumber with 2 tbsp of green goddess dressing
- **Dinner** Atkins Frozen Crustless Chicken Pot Pie; 1tbsp of olive oil and ½ cup of Brussels sprouts

Day 5

- **Breakfast** Atkins Frozen Cheese and Ham Omelet.
- **Lunch** Atkins Frozen Chili Con Carne with 2tbsp of Italian dressing and 2 cups of mixed greens.
- **Snacks** 2tbsp of ranch dressing with 1 cup of sliced red bell pepper and Atkins friendly Strawberry Shake.
- **Dinner** Cauliflower and Chicken Chorizo Sauté with sausage and cheese.

Day 6

- **Breakfast** Beef sautéed with onions and peppers topped with cheese.
- **Lunch** Atkins friendly Creamy Chocolate Shake
- **Snacks** Atkins friendly Caramel Chocolate Peanut Nougat Bar; 2 ounces of cheddar with 5 snap peas.
- **Dinner** Atkins friendly Frozen Beef Merlot.

Day 7

- **Breakfast** Atkins friendly Chocolate Almond Caramel Bar.
- **Lunch** Cobb salad.
- **Snacks** 2oz cheddar with 2 celery stalks; 2tbsp of ranch dressing with ½ cup of chopped red bell peppers.
- **Dinner** Portobello Mushroom Gravy with Atkins Frozen Meatloaf.

Here's what a week of eating could look like on the Atkins 40 diet.

Day 1

- **Breakfast** Spinach and cheese omelet with salsa and avocado and a slice of a bread of whole grain.
- **Lunch** Stir-fried roast chicken.
- **Snack** ¼ cup of blueberries or handful of walnuts.
- **Dinner** Broccoli and chicken Alfredo and a salad.

Day 2

- **Breakfast** Atkins friendly chicken chorizo cauliflower sauté with salsa and cheese.
- **Lunch** Chicken and kale Caesar salad.
- **Snacks** Atkins friendly Milk Chocolate Delight Shake with ½ small banana.
- **Dinner** ¼ cup of wild rice with 6oz of salmon, 2 tbsp of peanut butter with ½ cup of sliced cucumbers and 2 cups of mixed greens.

Day 3

- **Breakfast** Atkins friendly Vanilla Shake.
- **Lunch** Atkins friendly Frozen Shrimp Scampi with a small tomato, 2 tbsp of Caesar dressing, 2 cups of mixed greens and ½ avocado.
- **Snacks** 1 small carrot with ¼ cup of hummus; ½ cup of Greek yogurt with ½ cup of blackberries.
- **Dinner** Cauliflower Mash and Chimichurri Steak which are Atkins friendly.

Day 4

- **Breakfast** Oatmeal topped with ¼ cup of sliced strawberries and ¼ cup of chopped pecans.
- **Lunch** 5oz hamburger, a medium tomato, an avocado,1oz of cheddar cheese and 2 small Bibb lettuce leaves.
- **Snacks** Atkins friendly Creamy Lemon Smoothie; 2tbsp of green goddess dressing and ½ cup of chopped green bell pepper with 1oz of feta cheese.
- **Dinner** 6oz whitefish with ¼ cup of lentils, 1tbsp of butter and 1cup of green beans.

Day 5

- **Breakfast** Atkins friendly Frozen Farmhouse Style Scramble of sausages.
- **Lunch** 6oz Atkins turkey cutlets, 1tbsp of butter, 2cups of mixed greens, ½ cup of sliced bell pepper, ½ cup of sliced cucumber and 2 tbsp of raspberry vinaigrette
- **Snacks** 2 celery stalks with 2 tbsp of feta-ranch dressing, an ½ small apple and 2 oz of cheddar cheese.
- **Dinner** Atkins friendly Pork Chops With Fresh Mushrooms, a Bell Pepper and tomatoes with a ½ small baked potato, 2 tbsp of sour cream and 2 tbsp of butter.

Day 6

- **Breakfast** Atkins friendly Breakfast Mexi Peppers
- **Lunch** Cucumber, Tomato and Onion Salad With 4oz of turkey salami and a Creamy Feta Dressing.
- **Snacks** ½ cup of avocado and 2 tbsp of Greek vinaigrette; ½ cup of medium pear and 1oz of Brie cheese
- **Dinner** 6oz chicken, ¼ cup of brown rice, ¾ cup of stir-fry vegetables, 1tbsp of olive oil and 1tbsp of tamari sauce.

Day 7

- **Breakfast** Protein Pancakes with Double Chocolate.
- **Lunch** Snap Peas with Can Tuna, tomato, ½ of wheat pita and a Red Bell Pepper.
- **Snacks** Atkins Peanut Butter Crisp Bar with ¼ cup of hummus.
- **Dinner** Atkins friendly Beef Stroganoff

Here's what a week of eating could look like on the Atkins 100 diet.

Day 1

- **Breakfast** scrambled eggs with bacon, a tomato, green bell peppers and half a whole-wheat bagel.
- **Snacks** Atkins friendly White Chocolate Macadamia Nut Bar; small apple with 1oz of cheddar cheese
- **Lunch** Atkins friendly, Frozen Meat Lasagna with ½ cup of sliced cucumber, two cups of mixed greens, 5 cherry tomatoes and 1 cup of shredded carrot
- **Dinner** 2 cups of steamed broccoli with a Popcorn Garlic Shrimp, a cauliflower and ½ cup of brown rice.

Day 2

- **Breakfast** A small banana and a Milk Chocolate Protein Muffin
- **Lunch** A Cauliflower and Macaroni Salad with 5oz of hamburger, a whole-wheat bun, 2tbsp of onions and 2 tbsp of barbecue sauce.
- **Snacks** Atkins friendly, Mocha Latte Shake; ½ cup of strawberries with 4oz of plain unsweetened yogurt.
- **Dinner** 6oz of chicken breast, ¼ cup of chickpeas, 2tbsp of Cajun Rub, ¼ cup of baked acorn squash, 5 cherry tomatoes, 2 tbsp of Blue Cheese Dressing and 2 cups of mixed greens.

Day 3

- **Breakfast** Atkins friendly Farmhouse-Style Sausage Scramble with ½ cup of cubed honeydew melon.
- **Lunch** Atkins friendly Frozen Chicken Marsala with 2 cups of greens, ½ cup of sliced red bell pepper and 2 tbsp of Parmesan Peppercorn Dressing
- **Snacks** Atkins friendly Dark Chocolate Royale Shake; 15 corn of tortilla chips with 4 tbsp of black bean dip.
- **Dinner** A small tomato, 6oz of flank steak, ¼ cup of shredded carrot, 2 tbsp of Barbecue Rub, a medium sweet potato, 2 cups of baby kale, and 2 tbsp of Maple-Dijon Dressing.

Day 4

- **Breakfast** Atkins friendly Frozen Ham and Cheese Omelet.
- **Lunch** Grilled Lime Chicken with Spinach Salad, Sweet Cherry Pie and Feta-Ranch Dressing.
- **Snacks** A large tomato with 4 tbsp of hummus, Atkins friendly Mocha Latte Shake with a small banana.
- **Dinner** Classic Coleslaw and Quick Barbecued Pork with ¼ of a whole acorn squash and a whole-wheat bun.

Day 5

- **Breakfast** French Toast Loaf with 10 pecan halves and ¼ cup of blueberries.
- **Lunch** Chicken Sandwich with salad, Walnuts and Grapes.
- **Snacks** Atkins friendly Peanut Butter Fudge Bar and a small apple, ½ medium cucumber and 4 tbsp of black bean dip.
- **Dinner** Atkins friendly Frozen Stone Fired Meat Pizza served with Almond-Cinnamon Meringues, 2 cups of mixed greens, ½ cup of sliced bell pepper, 2 tbsp of Garlic Ranch Dressing and 1 cup of chickpeas.

Day 6

- **Breakfast** Fresh Blueberry Sauce with Sour Cream Waffles.
- **Lunch** Atkins friendly Frozen Mexican style Vegetable and Chicken with ½ cup of wild rice.
- **Snacks** Atkins friendly, French Vanilla Shake; 1tbsp of cream cheese with ½ cup of whole-wheat bagel.
- **Dinner** Fresh Guacamole and Fajita Steak with ¼ cup of Salsa Cruda, two 6-inch of corn tortillas and ¼ cup of black beans.

Day 7

- **Breakfast** ½ cup of blueberries and Protein Powered Oatmeal.
- **Lunch** Celery Salad and Daikon with 3.2 ounces of Italian sausage link, ½ cup of Basic Tomato Sauce and 1 cup of macaroni.
- **Snacks** Atkins Dark Chocolate Coconut Crunch Bar and a small tomato with ½ cup of cottage cheese
- **Dinner** Atkins friendly Frozen Chicken with ½ cup of peas and ¼ cup of brown rice.

3.6 Atkins-Friendly Snack Ideas:

One may consume balanced, low-carb snacks as well. In the Atkins diet, often people find it like their hunger is going down. They appear to be more than pleased with three meals a day (sometimes only 2).

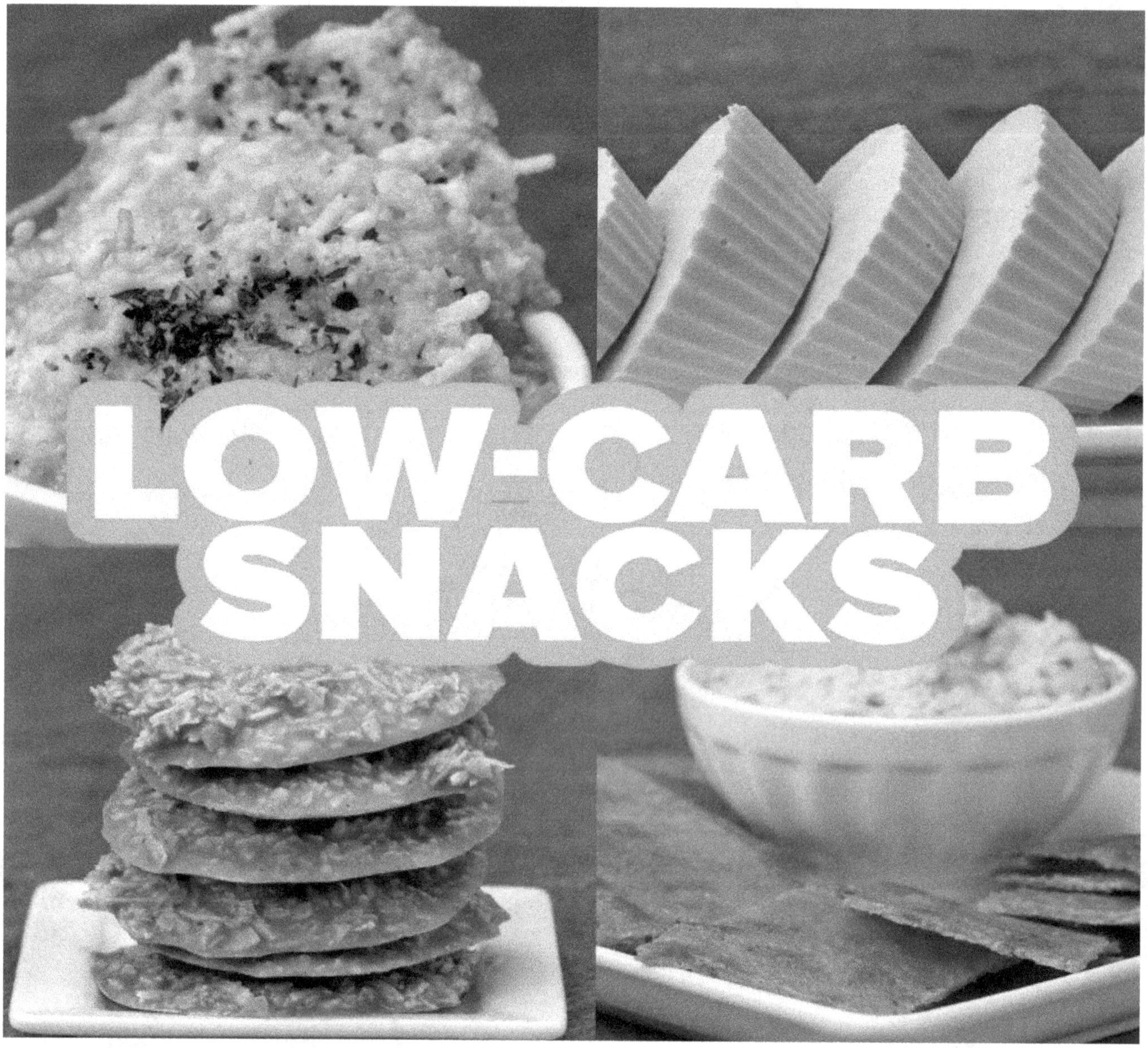

If you feel hungry later, however, here are a few quick, healthy snacks:

- A hard-boiled egg or two.
- Leftovers.
- A piece of meat.
- Berries and whipped cream.
- Fruits (after induction)

- A handful of nuts.
- Some Greek yogurt.
- A piece of cheese.
- Baby carrots (careful during induction).

If you are on the Atkins 20 diet, you can choose these snacks such as:

- Crab dip with vegetables
- Smoked salmon, cucumber, and cream cheese roll-ups
- Black olives with cheddar
- Kale chips
- Cucumber guacamole

If you are on the Atkins 40 diet plan, you can have any snacks such as:

- A slice of whole-grain toast with almond butter
- Hummus
- ¾ cup of blackberries
- Greek yogurt

If the regular net carbohydrates may not reach 100 g, the Atkins 100 plan followers can have any snacks.

You can steadily put back healthy carbs after induction is completed:

The Atkins diet is quite versatile, considering what you might have heard. You need to limit the consumption of carb sources only during the two-week induction process. After induction is done, nutritious carbohydrates such as higher-carb tomatoes, fruits, nuts, legumes, potatoes, and healthy grains such as oats and rice may be progressively added. However, even though you meet your weight reduction targets, chances are you may need to remain moderately low carb for life. You will gain the weight back if you resume consuming the same old things again in the same proportions as before. This is true in every plan for weight reduction.

3.7 What About Vegetarians?

Yeah, vegetarians and vegans can adopt the Atkins diet, but it would be more challenging to reach protein targets since certain go-to protein options are off-limits, such as seafood and beef (and milk for vegans). For all vegetarians and vegans, Atkins provides example menu plans and recipes, including carb totals.

If you are a vegetarian or vegan, you are going to start with extra carbs. In phase 2, vegetarians are given an additional handful, whereas vegans get about twice the normal amount of phase 2. (This is to get adequate nutrients from diets that could be more carb-heavy, in the absence of animal protein.) Most of your nutrition may have to come from plant sources (some vegetarians may even include eggs to make it easier), and you may need to include certain oils to boost your fat intake.

Researchers in Toronto created the Eco Atkins diet. 31 percent of calories come from (soy protein, eggs, tofu for vegetarians, veggie burgers for vegans, nuts, and cheese), 43 percent fat comes from (olive oil, avocado, and nuts), and 26 percent of the carbs from (fruit, vegetables, and whole grains). Small research conducted by BMJ Open in February 2014 showed that people lost around 15 lb. on the vegan version of the Eco Atkins diet after six months.

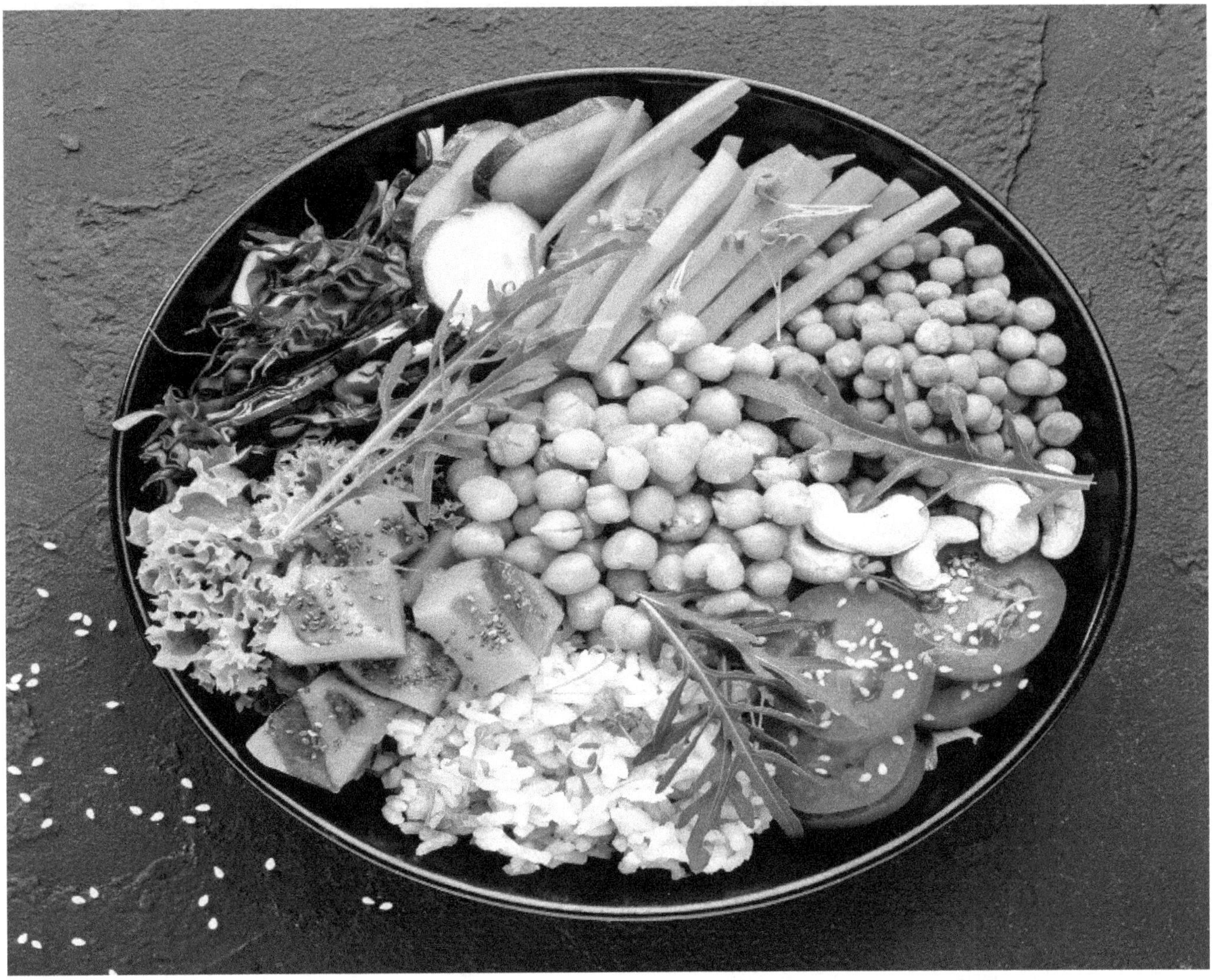

A multivitamin and a fish oil supplement (or flax oil for vegans) can both be used by vegans and vegetarians on the Atkins diet to guarantee that they receive sufficient amounts of nutrients. It is also advised that those on a diet leap straight onto Atkins 20 phase 2 or Atkins 40 as the Eco Atkins version's induction phase may be quite challenging. For Atkins, there is no need to add salt to all recipes. Stay well away from processed and dried foods as soon as you can, as sugar, other carbs and salt are sometimes added to them, which are bad for you.

Atkins does not require meat to be consumed by you. You are just going to have to skip the first phase of Atkins 20, which is too restricted to carbohydrates.

Vegetarians can get protein from:

- Eggs
- Eggs
- Nuts
- Legumes
- Cheese
- Soy
- Seeds
- High-protein grains like quinoa

Vegans can get protein from:

- Soy
- Nuts
- Legumes
- High-protein grains like quinoa
- Seeds

As a vegetarian (and vegan), it is possible to do the Atkins diet, however difficult. You should consume lots of nuts and seeds and use soy-based foods for protein. Excellent plant-based fat forms are olive oil and coconut oil. Lacto-ovo-vegetarians could also consume eggs, cheese, bacon, other high-fat dairy, and heavy cream.

Chapter 4: Easy To Make Recipes At Home:

The following are 7 Low-Carb Recipes in Under 10 Minutes:

The recipes below are easily prepared in less than 10 minutes, ideal for a busy, low-carb lifestyle at Atkins. There can be several health benefits from a low-carb Atkins diet, but you can struggle to create menu ideas that suit your busy schedule. It is simple to create delicious, low-carb meals that take less than 10 minutes of cooking time, even though you are not the most creative individual in the kitchen and have a few items at hand. All these meals are low-carb and friendly for weight loss.

- **Vegetables and Eggs Fried in Coconut Oil:**

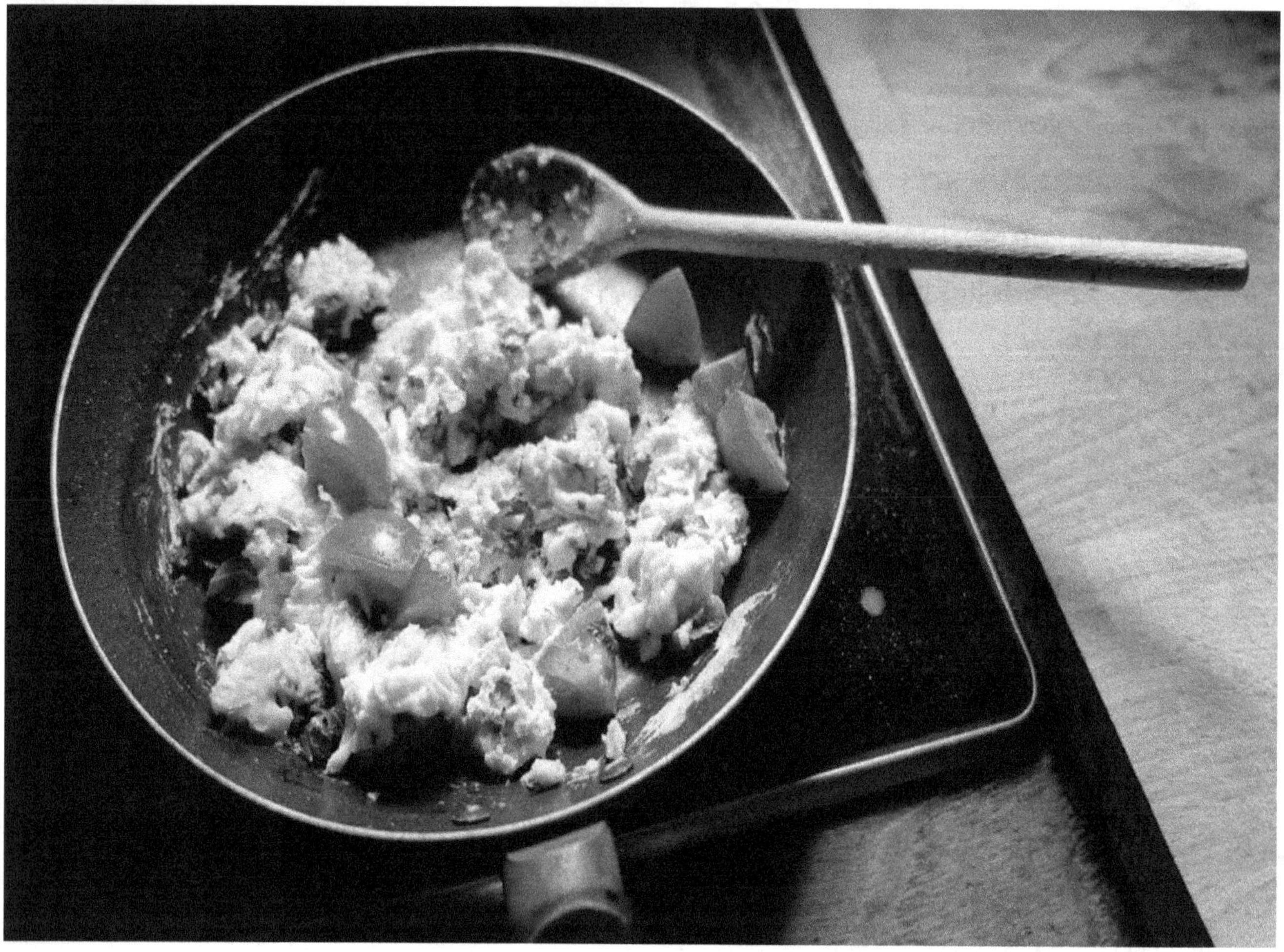

This meal offers a perfect breakfast for you to enjoy every day. It is abundant in nutritious veggies and protein and leaves you satisfied for a long period.

Ingredients: Fresh vegetables or a combination of frozen vegetables (carrots, broccoli, cauliflower, green beans), spices, eggs, spinach (optional) and coconut oil.

The instructions:

1. In the frying pan, add some coconut oil and turn on the heat.
2. Only add vegetables. Let the vegetables defrost in the heat for a couple of minutes if you have a frozen mixture.
3. Put in 3-4 eggs.
4. Add the seasoning, either a mixture of spices or only salt and black pepper.
5. Now add some spinach (optional).
6. Stir-fry until prepared.

- **Grilled Chicken Wings served With Salsa and Greens:**

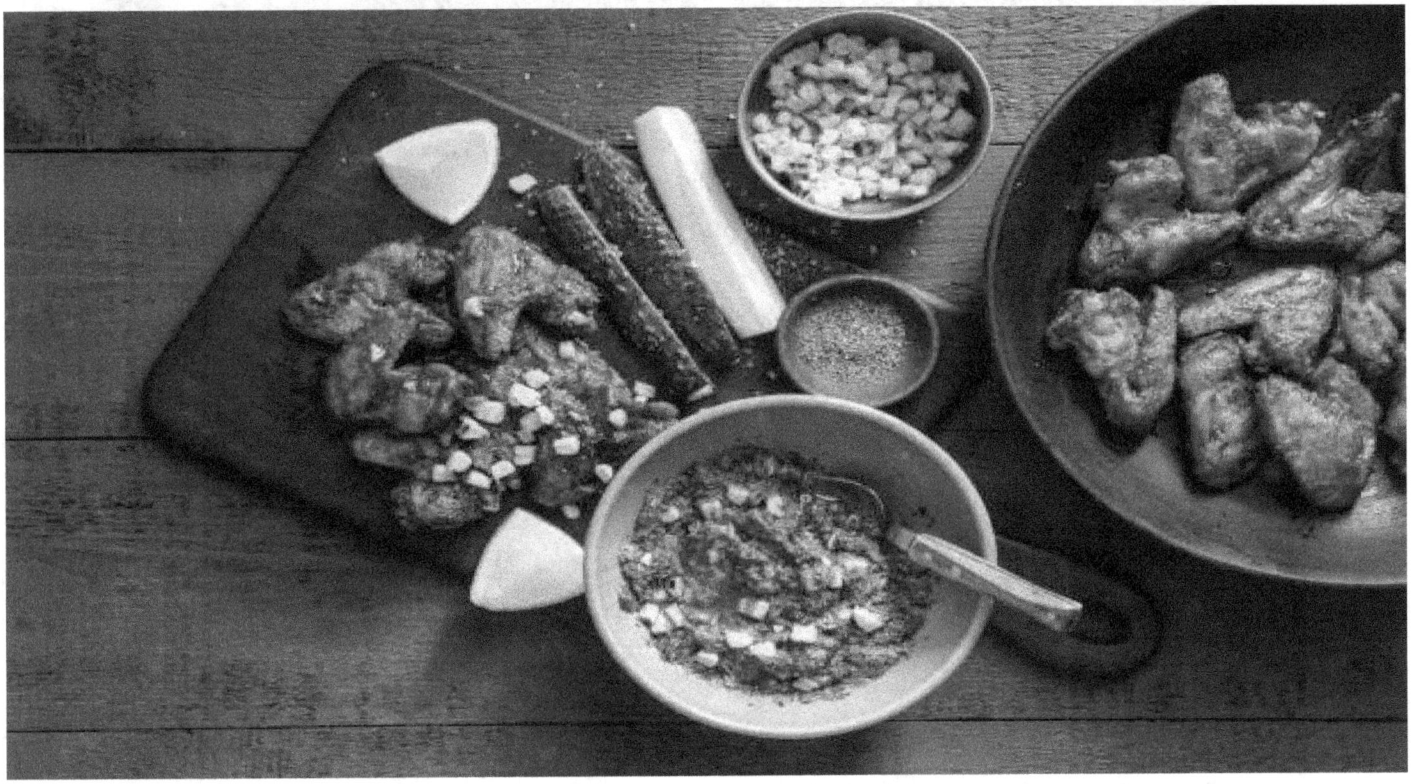

One of your favorites might just become this one. It needs little preparation because most people prefer to eat meat right from the bone. You might also find it meets the approval of your child.

Ingredients: Wings of chicken, peppers, salsa, greens.

The instructions:

1. In a seasoning mix of your choice, rub the chicken wings.
2. Put them in the microwave and heat them for around 40 minutes at 360-395 °F (180-200 °C).
3. Grill until the wings become crunchy and brown.
4. Serve with salsa and some greens.

- **Eggs and Bacon:**

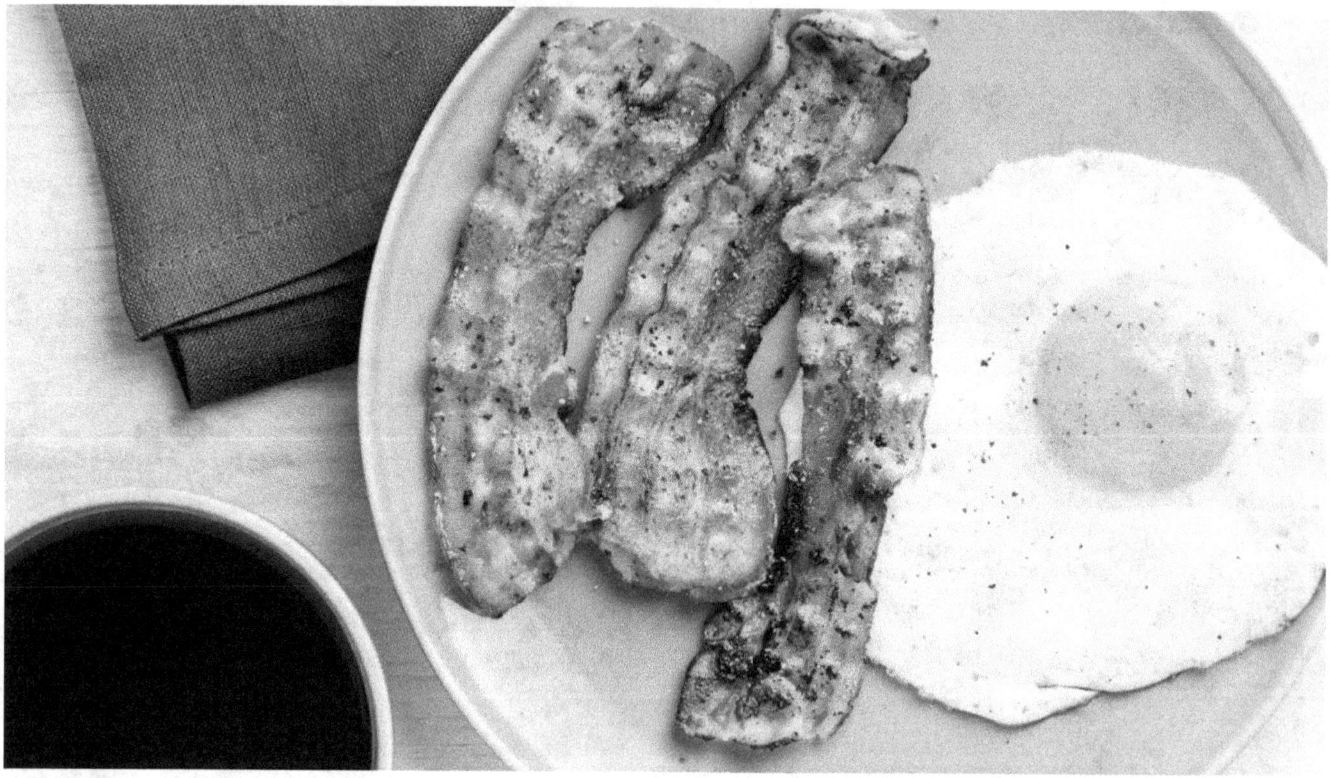

Although bacon is a meat that has been processed and is not exactly nutritious, it is low in carbs. In a low-carb diet, you can eat it and yet lose weight. There is nothing wrong with incorporating it into your diet if you maintain your bacon consumption in balance and do not consume it more than once or twice a week. **Ingredients**: Milk, pork, spices (optional).

The instructions:

1. In a pan, add bacon and fry until ready.
2. Place the bacon and fried 3-4 eggs in the bacon fat on a pan.
3. Put a little garlic powder, onion powder and some sea salt on them when cooking if you want to give more spice to your eggs.

- **Ground Beef With thick slices of Bell Peppers**:

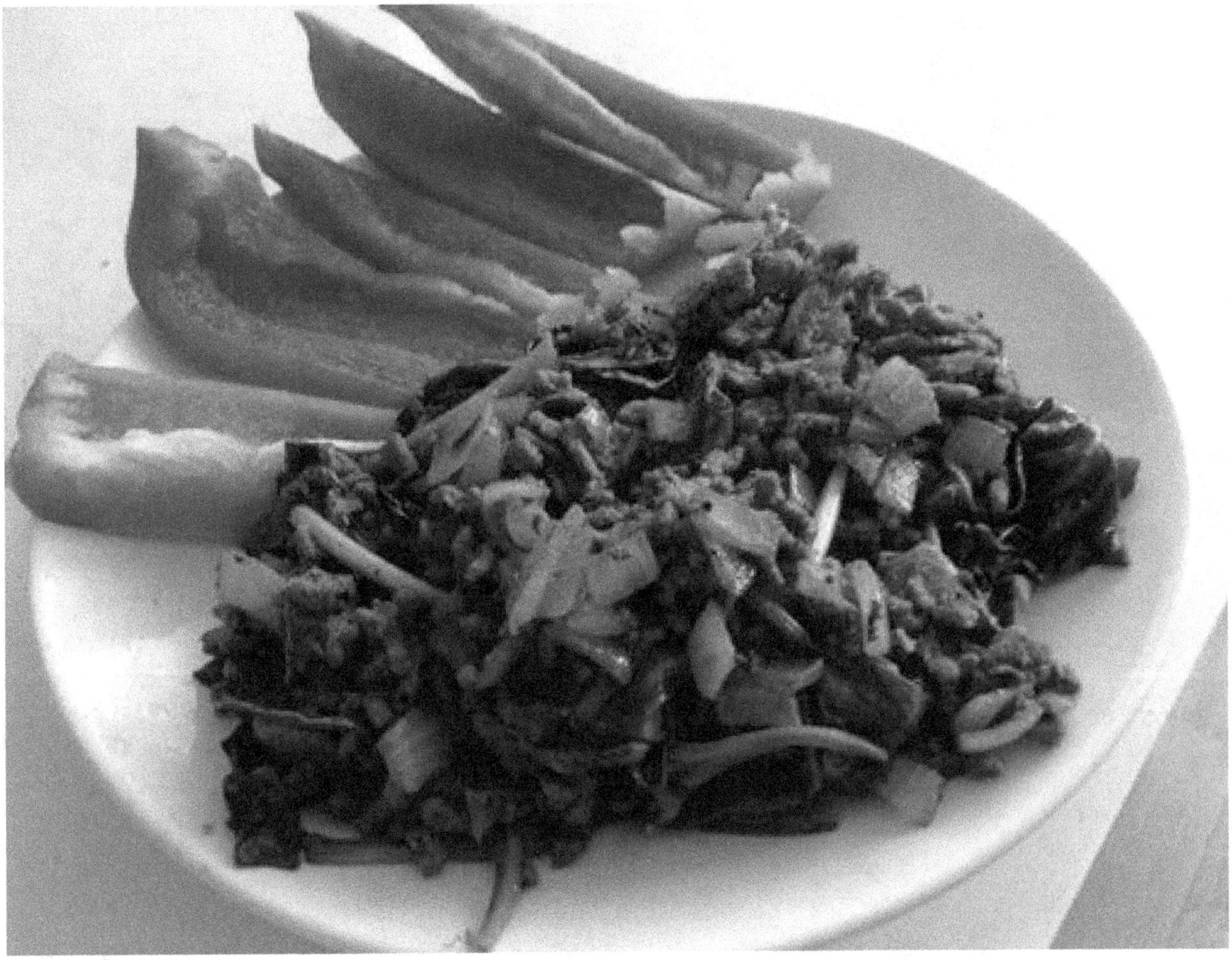

If you have some spare ground beef lying about, this low-carb meal is great.

Ingredients: coconut oil, ground beef, onion, herbs, bell pepper and spinach.

The instructions:

1. Chop the onion finely.
2. In a pan, add coconut oil and turn up the stove.
3. Add some onion, then stir for a minute or two.
4. Add some ground beef.
5. Add any of the ingredients, like a mix or just salt and pepper.
6. Now add some spinach.
7. You may add some black pepper and chili flakes if you like to spice it up a little.
8. Stir-fry and serve with sliced bell pepper when prepared.

- **Cheeseburgers without buns:**

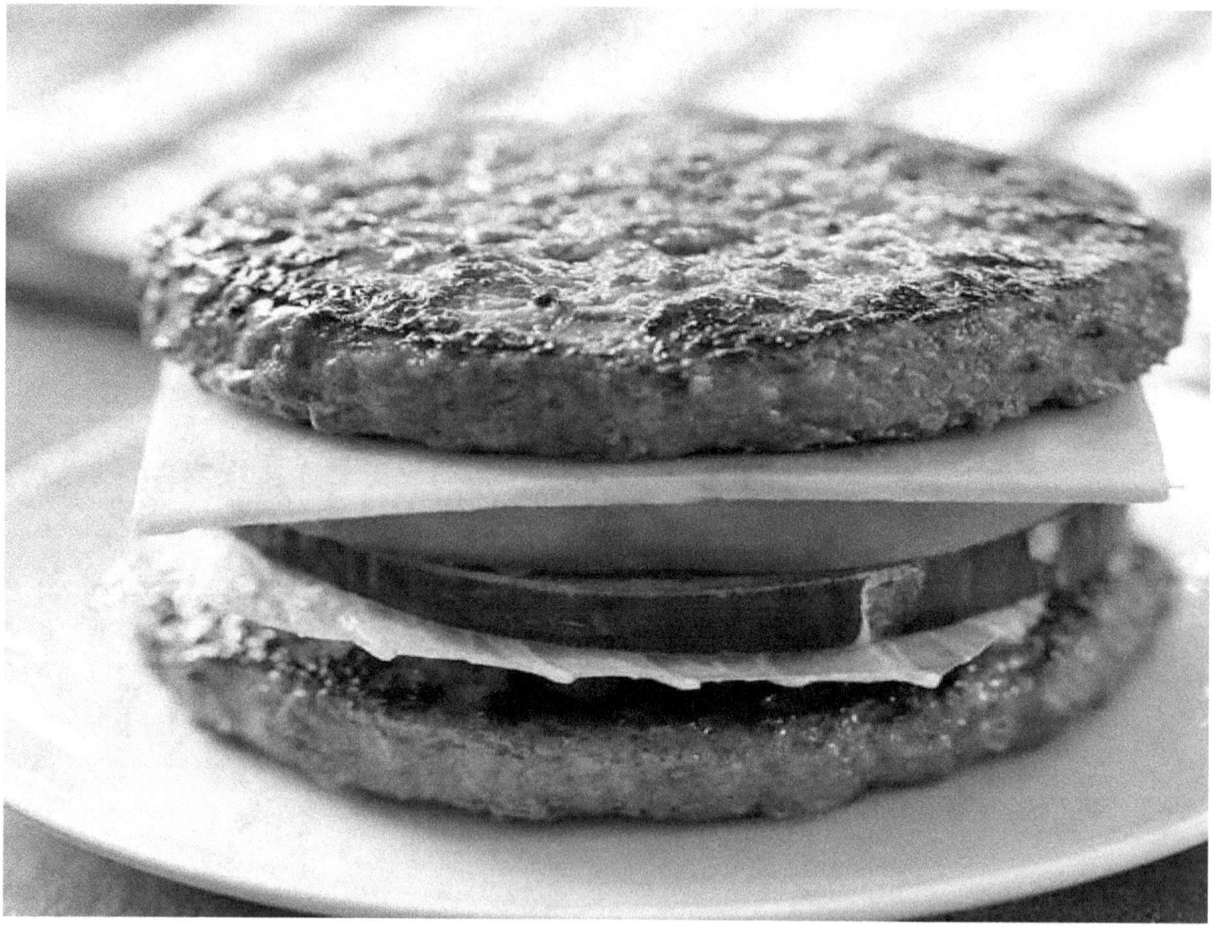

A bun less burger with two different types of cheese and a side of fresh spinach does not get any better than this:

Ingredients: Cheddar cheese, butter, hamburger patties, cream cheese, salsa, seasoning, spinach.

The instructions:

1. In a pan, add butter and turn the heat on.
2. Now add the hamburger patties and seasoning.
3. Flip the patties until they are nearly ready.
4. On top, add a few cheddar slices and some cream cheese.
5. Reduce the heat before the cheese melts and place a cover on the pan.
6. With fresh spinach, serve it. If you prefer, you can simmer some of the fats from the pan over your greens.
7. Add some sauce to make the burgers much juicier.

- **Fried Chunks of a Chicken Breast:**

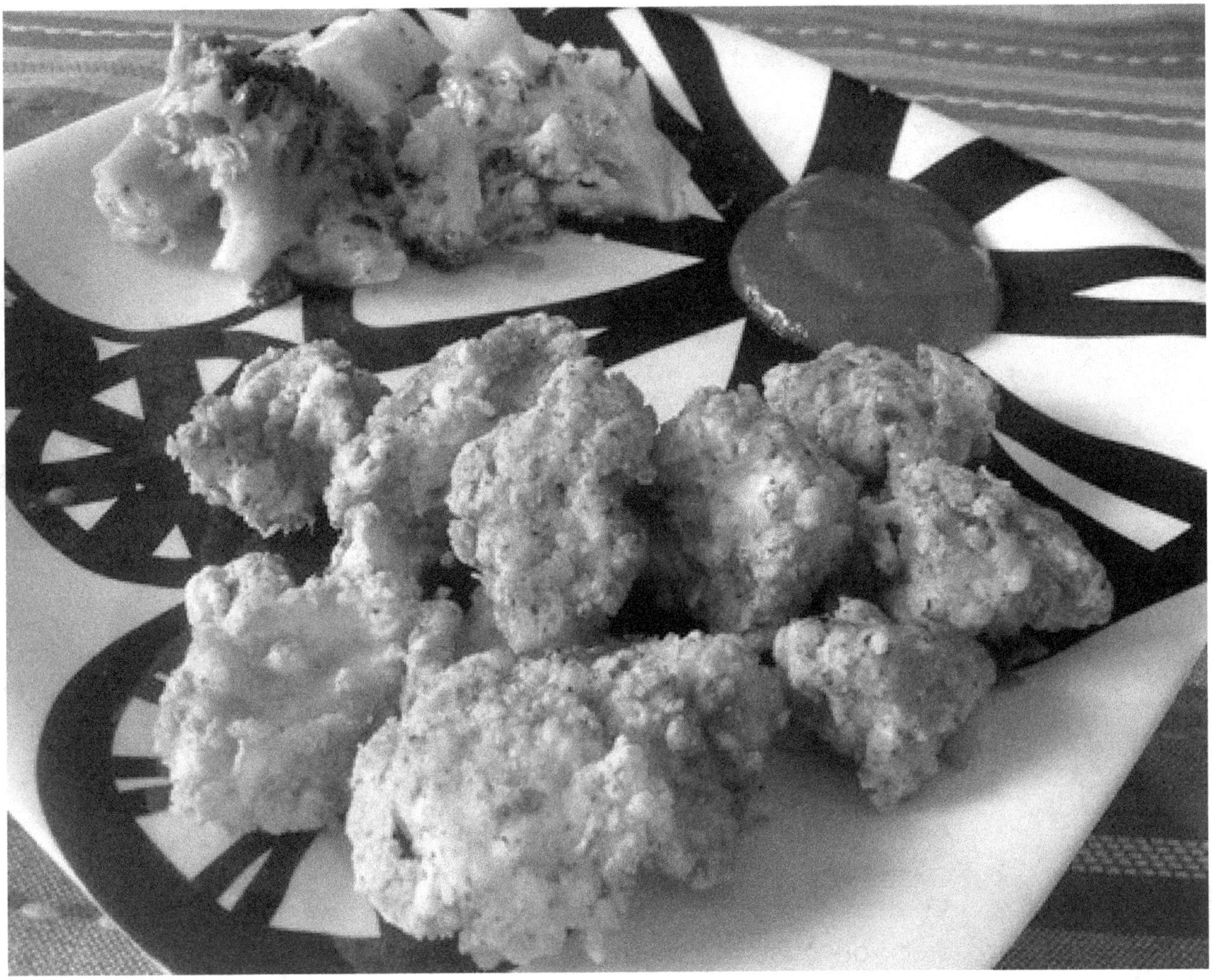

If you are nervous about ending up with distasteful, dry chicken and adding, some butter might be the trick.

Ingredients: butter, salt, chicken breast, spices, curry powder, garlic powder and leafy greens.

The instructions:

1. Cut the breast of the chicken into smaller pieces.
2. In a pan, add butter and turn the heat on.
3. Add pieces of chicken, salt, pepper, curry, and powdered garlic.
4. Brown the chicken till a crunchy appearance is reached.

5. Serve with some leafy vegetables.

- **Meatza, a combo of meat and pizza:**

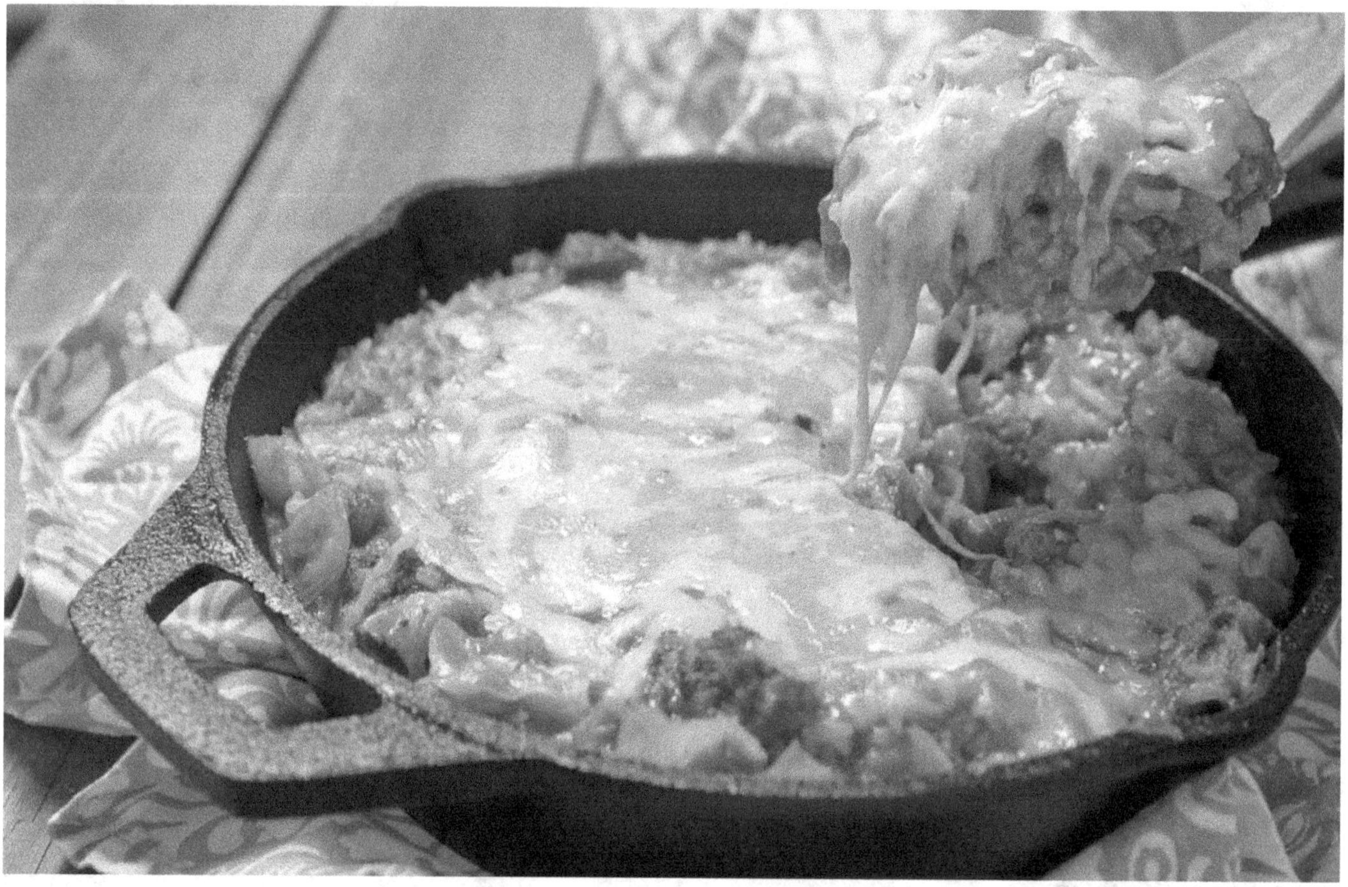

If on a low-carb diet you miss pizza, then you are going to love it. Without the harmful additives that many pizza types contain, you can find that it tastes much better. This recipe is simple to change, and you can add tomatoes, mushrooms, various cheeses, and any low-carb ingredients you like.

Ingredients: Sausage, tomatoes, ground beef, salsa, sauces, powdered garlic, and shredded cheese.

The instructions:

1. Chop the onions finely and slice some of the bacon into thin strips.
2. At the bottom of the baking dish, mix the ground beef, salsa, tomatoes, peppers, and garlic powder.
3. Sprinkle on top with melted cheese and layer with extra strips of bacon.

4. Put in the oven and heat for 30 to 40 minutes at 360 to 395 ° F (180 to 200 ° C) before the bacon and cheese look crunchy.

Chapter 5: Eating Out And Shopping With Atkins Plan:

It is entirely feasible to adhere to the diet when eating out with just a little planning. It is not important to eat organic, and always go with the least refined choice that suits the budget.

5.1 How to Follow the Atkins Diet When Eating Out:

Only because you are living a low-carb lifestyle does not imply that you need to avoid eating out to dinner every once and a while!

Ultimately, the safest diet for weight loss and other health issues is the one that a person practices to reach and sustain healthier body weight, so the Atkins diet is a strong and productive way to lose weight and stay healthy at the end of the day. You are not going to be disappointed.

When you think of beginning a low-carb weight loss diet, several people believe that it will eventually become a thing of the past to indulge in delicious food at their favorite restaurant. Not too easily! It can be just as simple, pleasant, and satisfying to eat out when on Atkins as before. Before you go out to dinner, consuming a light snack can help keep you from overeating at the restaurant. Pick food that is nutritious and filling, like vegetables and guacamole or a few turkey or ham roll-ups, but it will not ruin your appetite.

First, consider the genre of cuisine as you pick a restaurant. "Choose a restaurant that will serve more protein-based dishes than an Italian restaurant, such as an American restaurant," stated Rebecca Guterman, RD, a clinical dietitian at New York City's Mount Sinai Hospital. Before you arrive, check the menu online so you can plot your order in advance. Look for recipes that rely on lean meats and veggies. A salad served with grilled chicken or a burger without a bun, and a side salad is a decent choice. In place of bread, rice or potatoes, some suggestions include getting extra veggies. Order a meal typically based on fatty meat or fish that is fatty. With your meal, get some extra sauce, butter, or olive oil.

Usually, implementing the Atkins diet at most restaurants is simple.

- **Start with salads:** Be conscious of the salad's ingredients; do not buy salads that come in a shell (such as taco salad) and go easy on add-ins like coleslaw and strips of tortilla. Also, make sure that every meat you get is grilled, not breaded, with your salad. When you are in the early stages of a low carb diet, fruits such as grapes and mango higher in carbohydrates are often avoided.

  Vegetables are low in net carbs and filled with fiber, ensuring that every meal is a perfect start. "Before your main entrance, always have a salad first, with greens and you will stop over doing it." Monica Patino lost about 46 pounds on Atkins.
- **Bring your own dressings with you:** Many people carry their favorite spices or small bottles of hot sauce with them, and when they eat out, spice their restaurant meals as desired. Take your sauce with you with your salad anytime you head out to a restaurant because you know just how much carbohydrates **you receive. Only take an old bottle and fill it in your purse** or pocket with your favorite dressing. Yeah, you might get an odd look, but it is worth the looks you will get when you are slim, stated Terry Elkins, who lost 103 pounds on the Atkins diet.
- **You know your triggers so try to avoid them.** Make a strategy in advance for how to prevent your meal from potential carb-filled pitfalls. And stick with that. "Dining out at Atkins is so convenient. You know what you should have right now and what a food trigger is. Do not feel guilty calling for broccoli or Brussels sprouts to supplement the fries or potatoes. I tell continuously,' Kindly keep the croutons.' You have got to do what you have got to do.' Stated Andrea Morgan, who lost 105 pounds on Atkins diet plan.
- **Request a substitute:** Restaurants are in the business of providing service. One can be more than able to satisfy most demands, as long as you are respectful to the server.

Do not be afraid to inquire about replacing things or getting it made as you like it when you dine out! Instead of fries or extra vegetables, I still ask for a salad in place of chips or pasta. Many restaurants can satisfy the order of a customer! Stated Emelie Jurgens (Lost 89 pounds). Several restaurants give free bread or baskets of tortilla chips to start the lunch. If you have a hard time avoiding the break basket temptation, kindly inform the server that you do not require the basket or inquire if necessary, for them to take that away earlier than usual. If salsa, hummus, or guacamole arrives with bread or chips comes with hummus, salsa, or guacamole, ask for its replacement.

- **Master the art of fast food:** Due to crazy job schedules, after-school activities and more, you can find yourselves at the fast-food drive-thru more regularly than you want. Cut back on your fast-food visits is not a bad idea, but if you go, there are choices. With respect to dining out, I have three little children who enjoy fast food. I have grown to enjoy Wendy's because they have no difficulty making a double hamburger without even a bun and encouraging me to replace French fries with a Caesar side salad. "My children remain happy, and I can stick to my plan." stated Randy Fisher who Lost 80 pounds while following Atkins diet.
- **Stay hydrated:** Often, hunger will stimulate thirst. And even a quick snack would also quench some food, causing hunger pangs until you head out to dinner. Grab and consume a huge quantity of water and get a string of cheese or unsalted walnuts or peanuts. Still remember the nutritious quality and fiber, but 2 to 4 net carbs are present in certain mini low-carb nuts. Cheryl Lynn Wolf appeared to have lost 50 pounds on Atkins diet.
- **Be adventurous:** Get creative with the restaurant menu and choose fresh low-carb items that you might never have eaten before. We still ride a fair deal, and that is when you choose to make your food options more adventurous. You can truly enjoy a grilled rack of lamb at a restaurant. It is better to pick the lower-carb options rather than a higher carb kind of bread, for example, whole-wheat bread. Such items as gravy are generally avoided and should be extremely careful about sauces, but you must trust that it is the best choice.

At some famous restaurants, here are a few low-carb dishes you can try:

- ✓ **Chili's** Chicken or Steak Fajitas without tortillas and toppings and with a double serving of vegetables instead of rice.
- ✓ **Olive Garden** Herb-Grilled Salmon with Parmesan garlic broccoli on the side

- ✓ **The Cheesecake Factory** Pan Seared Branzino with Lemon Butter
- ✓ **P.F. Chang's** Shrimp with Lobster Sauce
- ✓ **Butternut Squash Noodles** All you need is a little parmesan and olive oil on top.
- ✓ **Antipasto-Stuffed Chicken** This super simple chicken dinner can boast an absolute knock out of flavor.
- ✓ **Burrito Zucchini Boat:** Less carbs but more meat.
- ✓ **Zucchini Lasagna Roll-Ups** Your low-carb lasagna dreams have come true.
- ✓ **Mashed Cauliflower** You will not even miss the potatoes.
- ✓ **Taco Tomatoes** These are the prettiest low-carb tacos you will ever see.
- ✓ **Zucchini Sushi** These little bites are super refreshing.
- ✓ **Low-Carb Pot Pies** Rice with cauliflower makes a healthier pot pie crust.
- ✓ **Caprese Zoodles** The Caprese salad your life has been missing.
- ✓ **Chicken Parm Stuffed Peppers** There's no wrong way to eat chicken parm...but do try this way as well.
- ✓ **Eggplant Lasagna** This is the vegetarian lasagna you have been searching for.
- ✓ **Cheesesteak Stuffed Peppers** A Philly favorite with a twist!
- ✓ **Grilled Cabbage "Steaks"** These will let you think about cabbage in a whole new light.
- ✓ **Beef Zucchini Enchiladas** Low-carb enchiladas for the win!
- ✓ **Low-Carb Big Macs** The guilt free way to enjoy your favorite hamburger.
- ✓ **Zuddha Bowls** A low carb Buddha Bowl!

Avoid including condiments in the meal and go for extra veggies or side salad over a starchy side (honey, mustard, barbecue sauce and ketchup are cunningly high in carbs).

5.2 A Basic Atkins diet simple shopping list to follow:

Shopping on the perimeter of the store is a safe rule. This is a place typically where all the food is usually available.

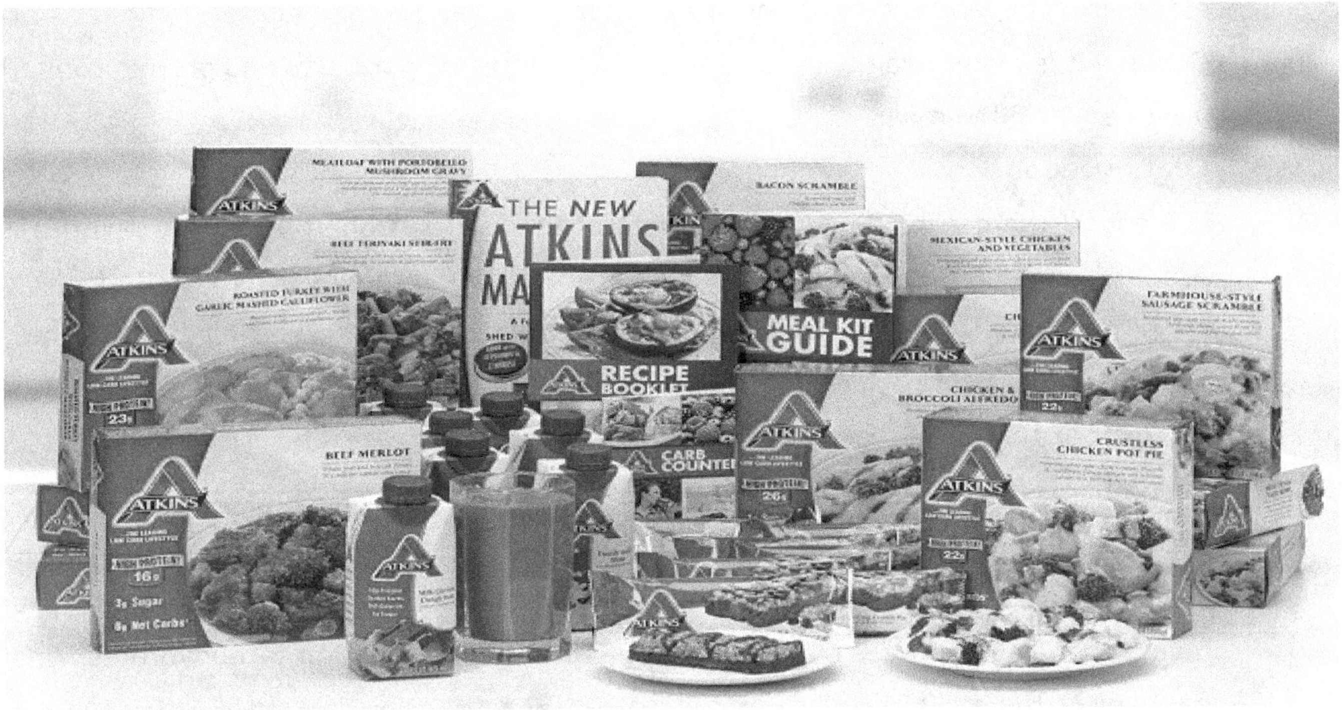

If you are preparing a diet for Atkins 20, Atkins 40 or Atkins 100, here are some important foods that you will need to buy:

- ✓ **Proteins,** including whitefish, chicken, pork chops, ground beef and salmon.
- ✓ **Vegetables** like broccoli, cauliflower, radishes, tomatoes, spinach, cauliflower, kale, lettuce, asparagus, onions, mushrooms etc.
- ✓ **Fats** like olive oil, butter, coconut oil and extra virgin olive oil.
- ✓ **Fruits** like pears, apples, oranges, and avocados.
- ✓ **Full-fat dairy products** like cheddar cheese, Greek yogurt, eggs, dressing of blue cheese, cream, eggs, and Greek yogurt.
- ✓ **Fatty fish:** Trout, salmon etc.
- ✓ **Shellfish and Shrimp**.
- ✓ **Nuts:** Almonds, walnuts, macadamia nuts, hazelnuts, etc.
- ✓ **Seeds:** Pumpkin seeds, sunflower seeds etc.
- ✓ **Condiments:** Turmeric, pepper, garlic, cinnamon, parsley, sea salt etc.

  In the Atkins shopping list to adopt, the descriptions of certain widely valued nutritional products suggested by some nutritionists are:

- ✓ **Eggs**

  Compared to other diet plans, the Atkins diet embraces the whole egg that promotes low-fat egg whites as a protein-rich breakfast choice. That is because the yolk offers the body the requisite fats for the plan to run properly. slice half an avocado, drizzle extra virgin oil, add a sprinkle of sea salt, and then add a fried egg on top," says Dr. Cohen. "It is tasty, healthy, and simple. The mixture of good fats and protein convert it into a satisfying meal.

- ✓ **Leafy greens**

  "I'll eat all the greens for lunch, and lots of them," Dr. Cohen says. "My favorite is Arugula." Spinach and kale, since they are rich in vitamins C, k and A, and other nutrients, both are good options. So, eat as much as you can; these leafy greens are the best choice.

- ✓ **Cucumbers**

  Cucumber is technically a fruit, quite low in calories and a strong water quality, which tends to fill a person up. Eat cucumbers as a snack or as a topping for salads. The seeds can also be scooped out and you can make cucumber boats loaded with your favorite topping approved by Atkins. Notice when you quit eating carbohydrates, what happens to the body.

- ✓ **Salmon**

  Trader Joe's provides wild, already cooked Pacific salmon. Throughout the day, I will select this or flake it on top of a salad,' says Dr. Cohen. Salmon is rich in omega-3 fatty acids and proteins, and you can get the extra value of calcium from the edible if you prefer the canned one.

- ✓ **Peppers**

  Bell peppers are rich in fiber and vitamins. Stuff these peppers with a mix of cooked protein, such as pork or chicken, and vegetables, like onions, greens, garlic, or fresh herbs, to make an Atkins-approved meal. Then bake them in an oven with virgin olive oil sauteed on top of them.

- ✓ **Beef**

  While several low-calorie diets reject beef for leaner chicken or turkey, its higher fat content is accepted by the Atkins diet. "I like to get grass-fed beef and make a creative side dish with butter and sea salt, like mashed cauliflower," Dr. Cohen says.

- ✓ **Tuna**

Tuna is rich in protein and healthy fats, whether fresh or canned, making it one of the most enjoyable Atkins diet products. "Once a week, I will make canned chunk of light tuna-it has less mercury than white tuna," says Dr. Cohen. Dollop it on the lettuce, or dip it in with celery sticks, carrots, cucumber, or other favorite veggies.

✓ **Pickles**

Pickles are a perfect Atkins snack; before purchasing, be sure to review the sugar and salt quality. " Do not buy butter and bread pickles. They are soaked in sugar," says Dr. Cohen,

✓ **Chia seeds**

Chia seeds, tiny but strong, are a gold mine of protein, fiber, and healthy fat. They also create a balanced dessert that is Atkins-approved. "Chia seeds, half-and-a-half, monk-fruit sweetener, and some blueberries make pudding," Dr. Cohen states. The fats and proteins supply a sweet tooth with a satiating solution.

✓ **Cheese**

Yeah, cheese is listed in Atkins diet foods; moderation is the key. "I'm going to buy tons of veggies and make a huge salad with some protein and a little cheese on top," Dr. Cohen says. The particularly great option is blue cheese: it is so flavorful; you need a light sprinkling for a big flavor effect. Learn why these high-carb foods will ruin your health if you do not avoid consuming them.

✓ **Avocado**

You will also eat your favorite green fruit on the Atkins diet, Dr. Cohen assures you. Rejoice, avocado lovers. Healthy mono- and poly-unsaturated fats are filled in avocados that make you stay feeling full and balance blood sugar levels.

✓ **Asparagus**

Asparagus is a non-starchy vegetable, ensuring it will not add many net carbohydrates each day to your total. For a tasty side dish or salad topping, sauté it with garlic, extra virgin olive oil, lemon juice, salt, and pepper. These are the things consumed all the time by skinny people.

✓ **Broccoli**

Cruciferous vegetables such as broccoli, Dr. Cohen notes, are rich in fiber and low in carbohydrates, making them a better option for Atkins' diet foods. In the oven, bake them, or in a salad, add them raw to make your meal a satisfying one.

✓ **Full-fat dairy**

Load up on tofu and cottage cheese that are full in fat. You could also have whipped cream. "Berries are a good dessert with real whipped cream," says Dr. Cohen. Do not skip these other little improvements to your diet that will help you lose weight.

Clearing the pantry with all harmful items and products is strongly encouraged. It involves ice cream, bread, soda, beverages and baking products such as sugar and wheat flour and breakfast cereals.

Chapter 6: Typical Results:

Over the years, the Atkins diet plan has passed through several adjustments. There are several variables in the strict diet schedule that you can remember before implementing it. Atkins presents many advantages that may render it the best diet for others. But the disadvantages could rule it out for others. Whether you are considering this plan to lose weight for better, before you initiate the diet, make sure that you analyze both the pros and cons of Atkins.

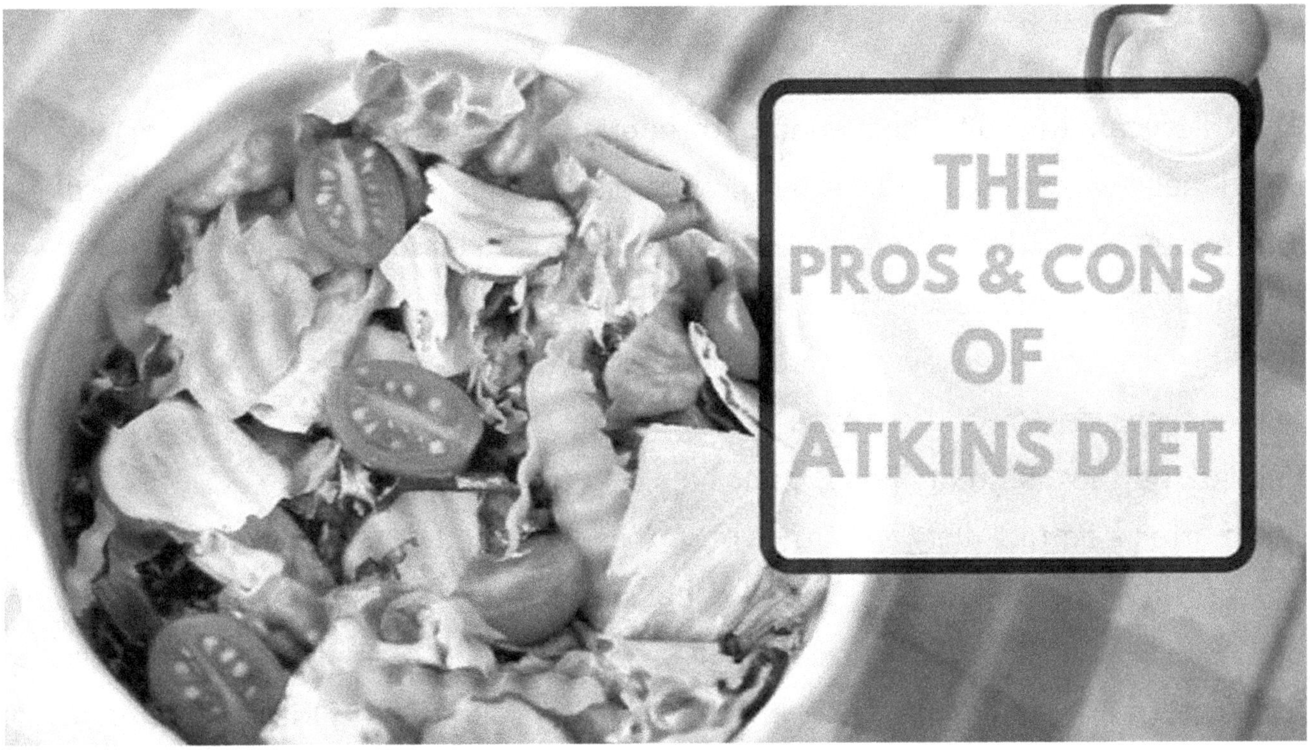

6.1 Pros and Cons:

The diet works on the idea that weight gain is induced by the metabolism of carbohydrates, particularly refined and starchy carbs such as wheat, potatoes, or pasta, not by fat consumption or food proportions, but by how our body system interacts the breakdown. The Atkins Diet includes a maintenance regimen for the first couple of weeks, which requires the incremental re-introduction of certain carbs into the diet to sustain weight loss. Even at this point, the carb consumption is far lower than most people are used to.

This diet can be quite challenging throughout the initial phase - especially for individuals who are used to large amounts of carbohydrates in their everyday diets. There can be a wide range of side effects from the dramatic fall in carb intake. Common ones are nausea, dizziness, migraines, and faintness in the first few days. Poor breath, triggered by the body heading through ketosis, is another somewhat unpleasant side-effect. For those who enjoy the thought of a fry-up each morning, The Atkins Diet is great. Eggs, pancakes, sausage, Baked, baked, grilled. It does not matter - on this diet, all of them are recommended. There are also very low to no carb ingredients in cheese, butter, and milk, and they are also advised on this diet. So, what do these topics all have in common? All of them are heavy in saturated fat, dieters are also cautious of whether it is appropriate to fill their bodies full of too much saturated fatty content.
There are also advantages and drawbacks of the Atkins Diet, as in other diets. This diet encourages accelerated weight reduction and requires dieters to ingest limitless fatty and protein-rich foods. This Atkins diet has also been found to not be as time-consuming and costly as some other common diets.
The Atkins Diet states that during the first two weeks of step 1, you will drop 15 pounds (6.8 kilograms), but it also admits that those are not standard outcomes. The Atkins Diet also admits that you will initially lose weight with liquids. It states that in phases 2 and 3, you can begin to lose weight as long as you are not eating more calories than your body will handle.

The Atkins diet will help an individual lose weight. For several, it would often lower the likelihood of type 2 diabetes, heart disease and would often lower other forms of metabolic syndrome by losing weight. Most people will lose weight, at least in the short term, with virtually every diet plan that limits calories. However, in the long run, findings indicate that low-carb diets such as the Atkins Diet are not any more successful than traditional weight-loss diets for weight loss and that, regardless of diet schedule, most individuals recover the weight they lose.

The primary explanation for weight reduction on the Atkins Diet is lower average calorie consumption by consuming fewer carbs because carbohydrates typically supply more than half of the calories eaten. Any reports indicate that the Atkins Diet has other causes for weight loss. Although the extra fat and protein keep you staying full longer, you will lose pounds, so your food options are reduced, and you consume less. These two effects lead to lower average consumption of calories.

PROS:

Weight Loss	Up to 15 pounds in the first two weeks (including water weight).	water
Food	Low-carbohydrates, high-fat commercial plan.	
A healthy Heart	May lower blood pressure, raise good cholesterol.	

It may be a perfect way to drop more weight and improve the overall health to follow a diet, but there are more precise factors why everyone chooses a diet. That can include decreasing blood pressure or cholesterol levels, minimizing the risk for heart disease, or increasing energy levels. A handful of possible pros are available to follow the Atkins food schedule.

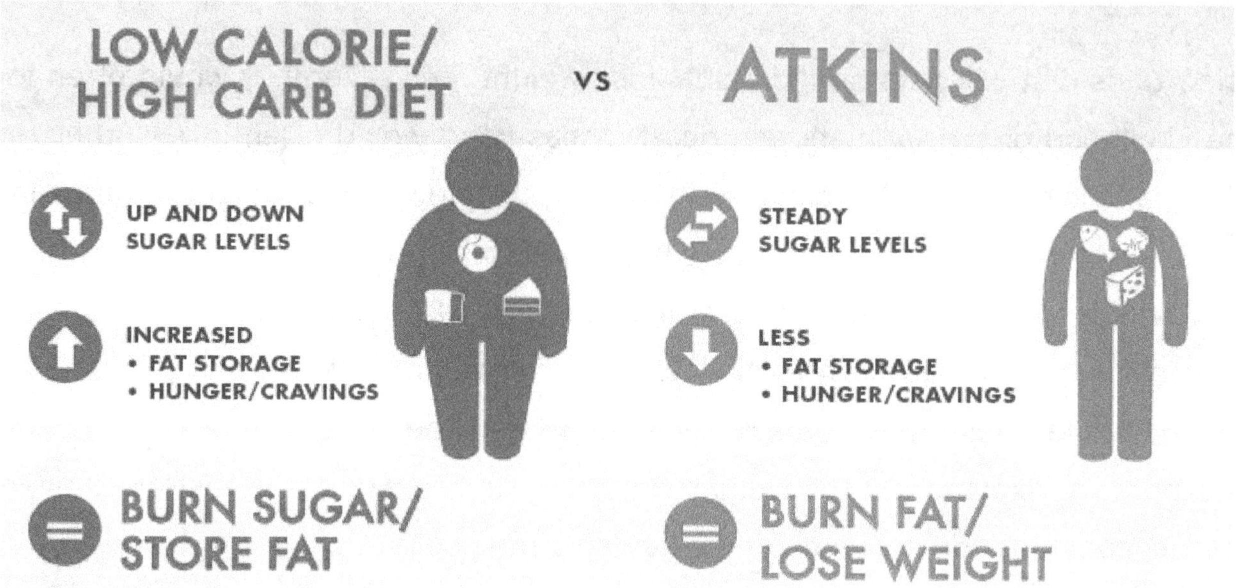
LOW CALORIE/
HIGH CARB DIET
VS
ATKINS
UP AND DOWN
SUGAR LEVELS
INCREASED
• FAT STORAGE
• HUNGER/CRAVINGS
BURN SUGAR/
STORE FAT
STEADY
SUGAR LEVELS
LESS
• FAT STORAGE
• HUNGER/CRAVINGS
BURN FAT/
LOSE WEIGHT

For one, the diet is reasonably simple to stick to. Richard D. Feinman, Ph.D., a biochemistry professor at the State University of New York Downstate Medical Center in Brooklyn, New York, and the publisher and former co-editor in chief of the journal Nutrition & Metabolism, argues that a carbohydrate-restricted diet minimizes this fight. Any meal is a fight for people who struggle with weight, a serious psychological burden. Clinical trials on Atkins and diets restricted to carbohydrates were performed by Dr. Feinman. The secure part of the diet is the protein that will give you more control over the war on food.

The diet is also not based on managing portions used in typical diets by certain individuals as a challenge. What does the regulation of portions mean? Self-control, because there's no good record for it,' Feinman notes. Small servings are great, so if you are still starving, you can eat another small portion with a low-carbohydrate diet. You will be out of luck on a low-fat diet if you are still hungry.

Susan Kraus, RD, a professional dietitian at Hackensack University Medical Center in New Jersey, says the Atkins diet's simple form would make it simpler for some people to adhere to it. "People feel it is easy to follow." she says, "You focus on a few food groups, you have flexibility in that you do not have to calculate food, and you do not feel deprived."

By following the low-carb fad diet, individuals with type 2 diabetes aiming for a solution for elevated blood pressure will also be helped. Reducing carbohydrates, either you lose the weight or not, has a health advantage. For example, a January 2015 report in Diet suggests that lowering carbohydrates can help treat diabetes and metabolic syndrome. If you participate in the Atkins diet, there is detailed literature documenting the consequences of focusing on a low-carb diet. Many of these published findings have confirmed the usage of the plan for weight loss and other health benefits.

The Atkins Diet claims that its dietary regimen will avoid or improve severe health conditions, along with metabolic syndrome, diabetes, blood pressure or heart failure. Almost any diet that helps you shed excess weight can minimize heart disease and diabetes risk factors or even reverse them.

Weight Loss:

There is a fine record of effective weight reduction on the Atkins diet. Many individuals on this initiative have lost weight, and the method has been tested in several clinical studies. But you can find that there are many trials with contradictory results whether you recommend Atkins for weight reduction or weight management. An examination of findings conducted in the journal Nutrients contrasted Atkins to 19 different diets without clear expectations for calories.1 The researchers noticed that the Atkins diet showed the best proof of the examined diets in achieving clinically beneficial short-term and long-term weight reduction.

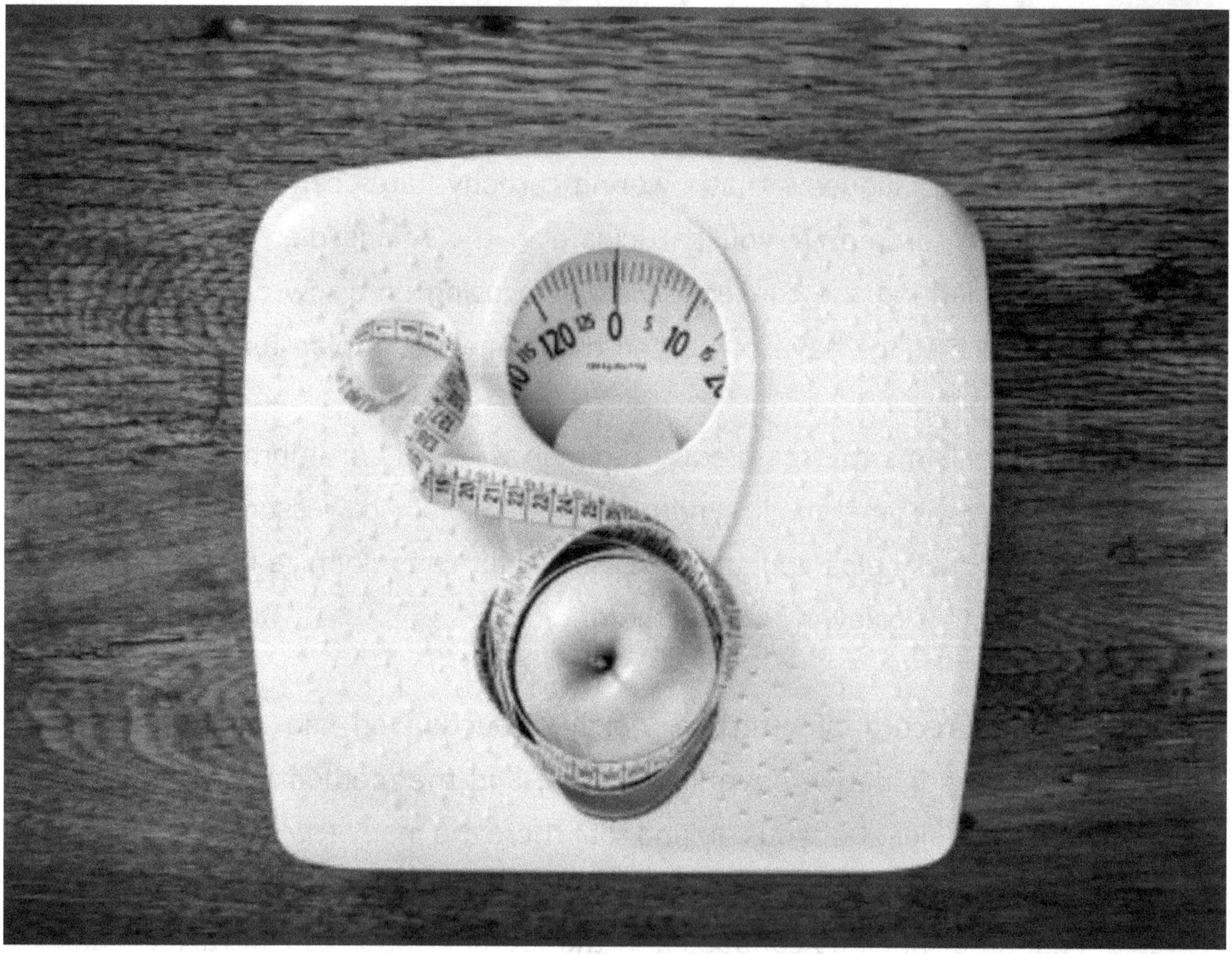

For two years, a further analysis conducted in the Annals of Internal Medicine examined 307 people. For two years, participants adopted either a low-fat diet or a low-carbohydrate nutrition program described in Dr. Atkins' New Diet Revolution. The study authors noticed that when combined with behavioral therapy, both programs could achieve substantial weight loss, but the low-carbohydrate approach was correlated with positive improvements in risk factors for cardiovascular disease. However, there is still an extensive study that compared high-fat ketogenic diets (like Atkins) to diets where there are limited calories. Many of these experiments have found that there is little distinction between calorie reduction and carb restriction for long-term weight reduction. Besides, while there is some encouragement for low-carbohydrate, higher fat diets, medical researchers are also debating whether the plan is safe for the long-term.

You may have chosen to start Atkins because you needed to lose weight, but did you realize that study has found that a low-carb diet like Atkins has shown far other advantages in 'off label' that only lose weight? These contain, to name a few: epilepsy and associated disorders, acid reflux (GERD), acne, headache, cardiac failure, cancer, polycystic ovary syndrome (PCOS), insulin resistance/diabetes/metabolic syndrome, dementia, and narcolepsy.

Epilepsy:

In certain patients on one or more antiepileptic medications, epilepsy is a debilitating and common neurological condition that can successfully manage. About 30 percent of people with seizures have refractory epilepsy, and correctly selected and utilized antiepileptic drug schedules have failed sufficient studies to induce prolonged relief of epilepsy.

More than 30 reports from 2004 to 2014 endorse the usage of a Modified Atkins Diet in adults and adolescents to better relieve the effects of epilepsy and associated seizure disorders. This has been extremely promising for children living with childhood epilepsy who do not respond to medication for seizure control.

A high-fat, low-protein, and carbohydrate diet, with few calories and fluids, consisting of the traditional Atkins diet, is a promising diet plan. The Atkins diet is a therapeutic modality that has been used as a treatment for intractable epilepsy since the 1920s. It has been suggested as a dietary therapy, which is already documented in the Hippocratic collection, that would produce similar fasting advantages. The Atkins diet is rich in fat and has minimal protein and carbohydrate content. Information suggests that for non-surgical Pharmacoresistant epilepsy patients of any generation, KD and its derivatives are a suitable choice, considering that the form of diet should be individually designed, and that less restrictive and more palatable diets are often safer choices for adults and teenagers. This analysis addresses the Atkins diet, including potential modes of action, applicability, side effects, and proof of its success and more palatable diets in children and adults, such as Low Glycemic index Diet (LGID) and the Modified Atkins Diet (MAD).

Control Diabetes:

Although most diets will help to overcome a broad variety of health conditions, the Atkins diet is the only option in our world today to address a particular and common medical problem: diabetes. 25.8 million persons in the United States (8.3 percent of the population) have diabetic issues, and 79 million individuals have pre-diabetes, as per the American Diabetes Association. This is a challenge that needs to be addressed seriously, with so many individuals now at risk for diabetes and the pace at which diagnosed cases are growing.

Weight reduction is one of the most key parameters of managing diabetes or maintaining health for a diabetic individual, and the Atkins diet is a perfect way to do this. The Atkins Diet is an excellent way to keep it from progressing, particularly though you do not have diabetes. Insulin resistance, or when their glucose levels do not want to go down, is what challenges certain individuals with type 2 diabetes. The trouble with insulin resistance is that the body system is slow to respond to the medication most likely to benefit it. This tolerance contributes to elevated insulin levels being prescribed to diabetics, and weight gain is a side effect of a high-level insulin treatment because insulin accelerates fat accumulation and synthesis. In brief, the harder someone do efforts to regulate their blood sugar level with insulin, the most possible it is for them to add weight.

What made the Atkins diet the best diabetic diet is that the amount of carbohydrates eaten is limited as the Atkins diet reduces the number of carbs consumed by a person. Although lowering calories can usually contribute to weight reduction, diabetic medications also cause side effects and appetite stimulation, rendering it impossible to lose weight on a normal diet.

Studies have shown that a low-carb diet will significantly increase blood glucose regulation and blood lipids for individuals with type 2 diabetes. These results are important since they offer a means for people with diabetes to minimize their obesity and treat their diabetes.

When you exclude added sugar and reduce the carb consumption to primarily 'foundation vegetables' while on the Atkins diet, insulin tolerance increases along with blood glucose regulation. Under the guidance of a specialist, several individuals who mainly eat foundation vegetables may notice that they will avoid or decrease their dependency on blood-sugar-lowering medicines. Before you are using Atkins, you can work very closely with the doctor to change the dosage. The need for medicine that reduces blood sugar would decline easily.

With your health and nutrition, one should be careful. There are tons of foods for diabetes, but the safest diabetes plan is the Atkins diet. If you have diabetes, or you are at risk of diabetes or wish to boost your overall health and lose weight, a perfect way to improve your health is to turn to the low carb Atkins diet and then focus on this healthy carbs diet.

The Atkins diet excludes processed carbohydrates like baked goods (such as cake and white bread) and supports the consumption of healthier carbohydrates, particularly in the later stages of the diet (such as green vegetables and berries rich in fiber). And you will understand the distinction between good and bad carbohydrates.

Simply lowering the consumption of processed grains and sugary drinks offers noticeable advantages for multiple individuals straight away. Instead of soda, consuming water and replacing starchy dishes with foundation vegetables are sure to benefit you, and you will have steady levels of energy during the day. Additionally, once you scale down on your carb consumption, you can drop water weight relatively quickly.

A healthy heart:

between 2002 and 2014, twenty-one studies examined the function of low-carb diets and how they may help reduce risk factors for cardiac disease and chances for depression and stroke. it has been demonstrated that the usage of a low-carb diet not only assists with weight control but often increases blood pressure, levels of cholesterol and triglycerides and reduces inflammation, these factors correlated with cardiac disease.

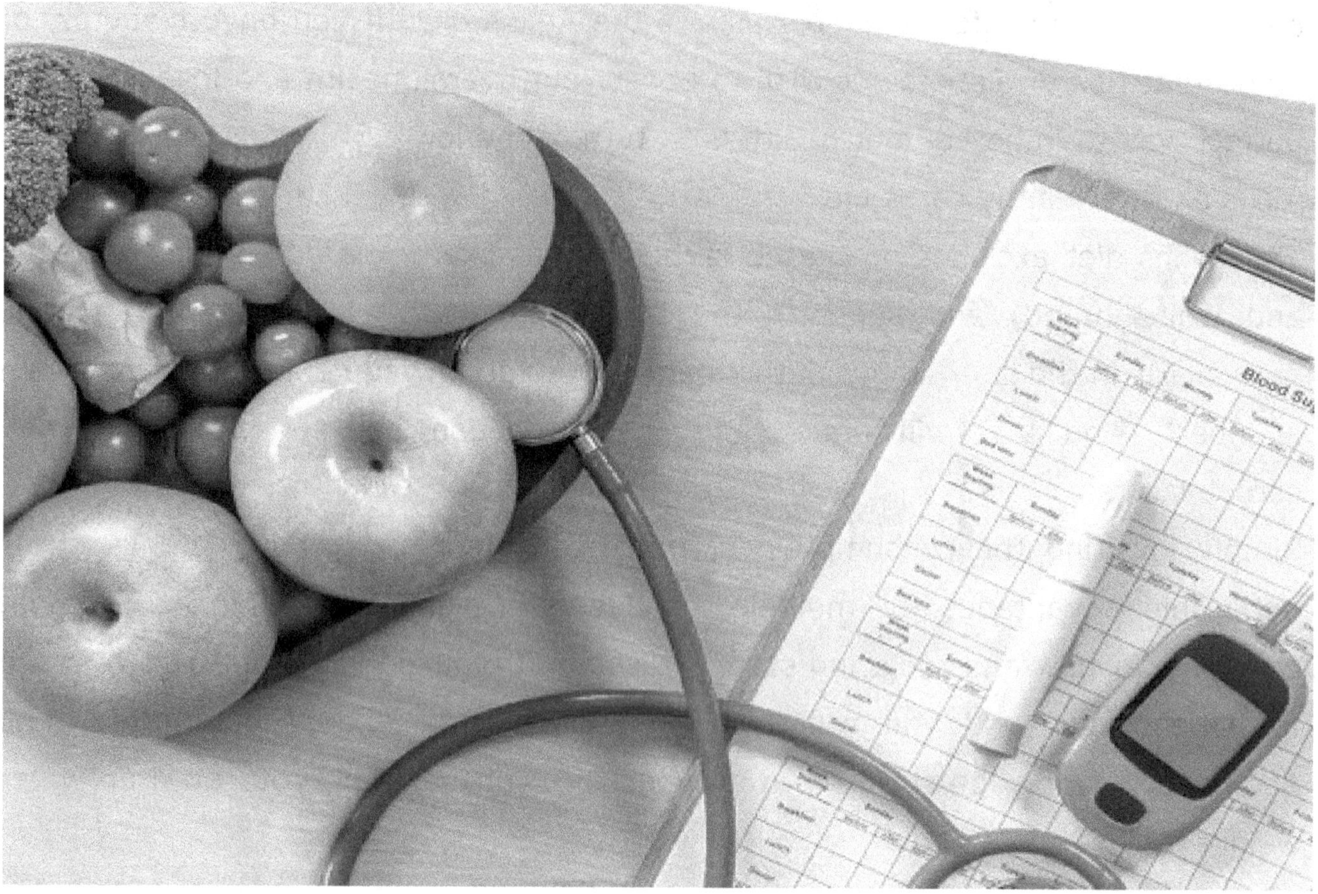

It is a sobering fact that the number one killer among Americans is heart failure. It is a vital opportunity to make sure you are doing all you can to keep yourself safe because February is American Heart Month. Any literature shows that Atkins improves healthy HDL cholesterol and reduces blood pressure, lowering the likelihood of stroke and heart disease. All that fat, though, scares most specialists. Some health professionals suggest that, as permitted on the Atkins Diet, consuming a significant amount of protein fat from animal sources can raise the risk of heart disease or some cancers, but thankfully, evidence continues to show that individuals who adopt a controlled-carb, higher-fat eating plan such as Atkins (which does not contain trans fats) typically have better amounts of 'good' HDL cholesterol and the lower number of triglycerides. They often lost more weight than people who adopted a standard low-fat diet. Some fats are healthy for your heart, and theyare essential components of Atkins, too. These fats include monounsaturated fats in almonds, avocados, olive oil, canola oil, and polyunsaturated fats found in seafood, soybeans, sunflower seeds and flaxseeds, and cottonseed, safflower oil and maize. Try to have fatty cold-water fish such as salmon, halibut, and tuna, high in omega-3 fatty acids, for at least two servings a week (3.5 ounces). Omega 3s can decrease triglycerides, slow down the atherosclerotic plaque rate, and lower blood pressure.

Cancer:

Obesity is a cause correlated with the elevated incidence of certain cancers, but a low-carb diet is seen to help people reduce weight and sustain their weight loss. It has a beneficial influence on lowering the risk of some cancers. an Examples involve results from a 2012 report in the Journal of National Cancer Institute indicating that higher average consumption of carbohydrates and higher dietary glycemic load is correlated with a high risk of recurrence and mortality in colon cancer in stage III, which suggests that a low-carb diet (which is super low glycemic) could help improve colon cancer survival rates. Another Nutrition and Cancer (2010) research found that a low-carb diet helps overweight women who are survivors of breast cancer reduce weight, lowering their likelihood of cardiac failure and other obesity-related illnesses, as well as breast cancer recurrence.

PCOS:

The most prevalent endocrine disease impacting women of reproductive age is polycystic ovary syndrome (PCOS) and is correlated with obesity, insulin resistance and hyperinsulinemia. since low carbohydrate diets have been shown to decrease insulin resistance, examined the six-month endocrine and metabolic effects of a low-carbohydrate, keto diet (LCKD) on overweight or obese women with PCOS in a pilot study (Nutrition and Metabolism, 2005). In this pilot study, in women with obesity and PCOS over 24 weeks, LCKD contributed to substantial changes in weight, LH/FSH ratio, percent free testosterone and fasting insulin. Another 2004 pilot analysis saw related promising findings in the Journal of General Internal Medicine showing resistance to Diabetes/Metabolic Syndrome/Insulin. Twenty-nine reports, going back to 1998, indicate that low-carb diets significantly reduce the effects and complications of diabetes, metabolic syndrome, and resistance to insulin.

No Calorie Counting:

Frustration with the use of counting calories for weight reduction and weight management is increasing. While most fitness experts understand the value of eating the correct number of calories per day, they recognize that it may be boring and restrictive to attempt and track and control your consumption every day.

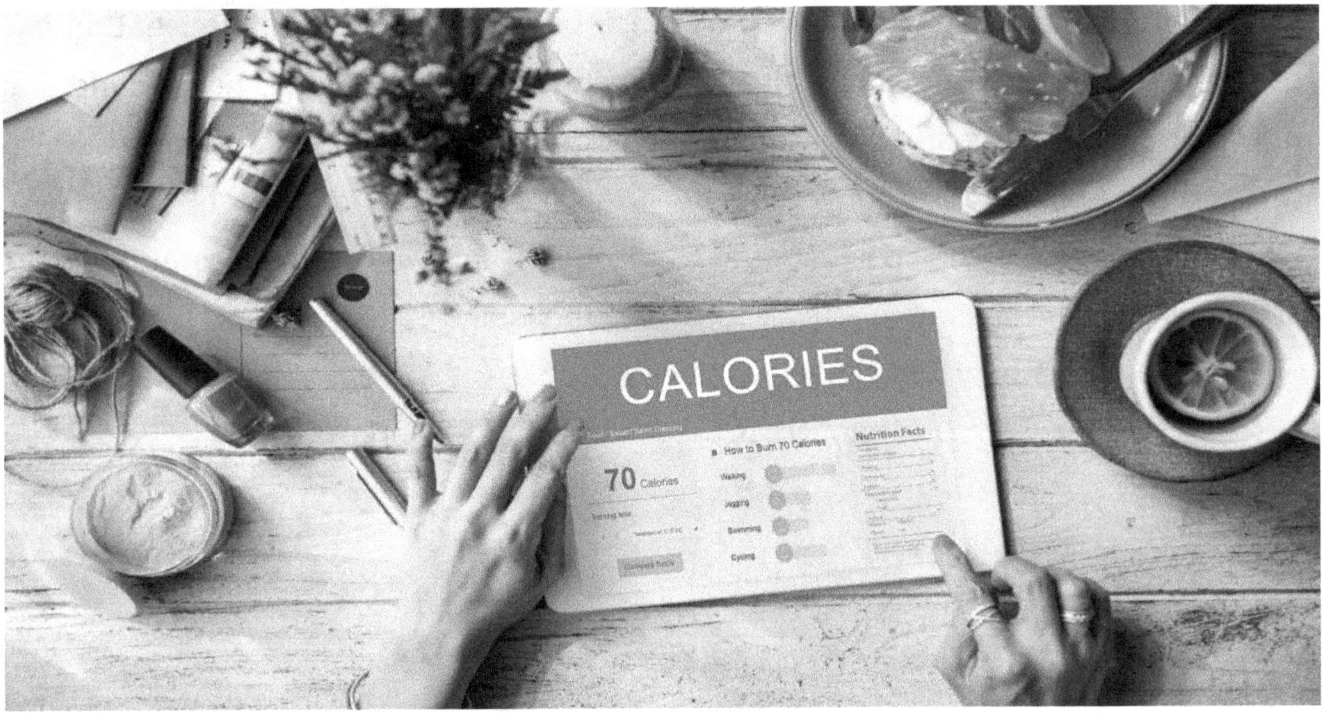

You track the Atkins plan's net carb consumption, so there is no requirement for calories to be counted or restricted. This aspect of the Atkins plan is the most attractive to many individuals.

Hearty Eating Plan:

Some people enjoy the idea that you will consume richer and fulfilling food on the Atkins diet schedule. Some may choose this diet, for instance, so hearty foods such as steaks and burgers will remain on their plate.

Foods high in protein and foods containing more fat seem to be more enjoyable. You are likely to postpone the next meal or snack because you feel full after eating and can consume fewer calories overall as a consequence. Several tests have found that the Atkins strategy has a lower average calorie consumption than other programs with a higher intake of carbohydrates.

However, it is necessary to remember that the more recent versions of Atkins have portion size guidelines. E.g., for added fat, the daily recommended consumption during Phase 1 is only 2-4 tablespoons. So, if you eat huge portions of fatty beef, butter, and cheese, you cannot trust the Atkins plan to work.

Clearly Defined Guidelines:

Atkins is enjoyed by many people who want a disciplined approach to food. Each phase of the plan has a particular duration or weight target that is specifically explained. Phase 1 lasts for two weeks, for example (in most situations). Until you become 10 pounds off your target weight, Step 2 lasts. Step 3 runs for four weeks before you are safely at your target weight. At each point, detailed lists of appropriate foods are available, and portion sizes for and type of food are specifically specified.

Anyone who has practiced Atkins will inform you about the advantages of a low-carb lifestyle; here are few unexpected advantages of dieting Atkins.

1. Willpower strengthens.

one can say, when you first think about Atkins, "How can I live without ice cream or bread?" Or some high carb snack that people enjoy. This all changes while following Atkins after a week or two. The cravings disappear when the blood sugar normalizes. In reality, if you have a 'blip' and consume any high carb junk, then you start to know how it makes you feel bloated and hungry. Plus, you are discovering new favorite recipes that nourish the body without zapping the life out of it.

2. Tell goodbye to hunger.

As Atkins diet conjures up visions of countless plates of lettuce, egg white omelets or worse, nothing, one does not want to think of Atkins as a 'diet.' This low carb, high protein plan leaves you feeling happy.

The truth, though, remains that people are too full to eat, but the pounds are coming off, and they feel fine. The reasoning for this is that, of course, each Atkins meal is high in protein and dietary fat, so it is really enjoyable, and you feel nicely satisfied because you are not cutting back on calories.

3. One can feel more focused:

You send a kid a bag of candy, and just before your eyes, you can see them becoming hyper. When they jump off the wall on a sugar high, they find it hard to concentrate on one thing.

Well, if the body transitions to ketosis, the inverse happens. You realize your mental concentration significantly enhances. This is a great advantage to Atkins that most individuals appear to lower their carbohydrates in a week or 2.

4. Enhances Stamina:

You can expect to see a significant rise in strength levels on a low carb diet once you have finished the adaptation period to move to ketosis (approximately 1-2 weeks). You will be motivated to raise more weights or realize you have more stamina to keep up with the kids. Exercise would be much easier. This is because, for nutrition, the body adapts to burning fat. Because we have a far higher abundance of fat than carbohydrates, energy levels are soaring. However, if you notice that after two weeks on Atkins, you are deficient in energy, try increasing salt consumption. Atkins is usually a diuretic, suggesting that as the water retention reduces, you must replace the lost salt. However, do not worry; you do not consume fatty, processed foods on Atkins to lower your consumption.

5. Your mood is dramatically change:

You will find that you feel a lot brighter without the frequent peaks and drops of blood sugar that zap vitality and steal your mood. When it comes to mind, diet serves like therapy because, although you might have already consumed sugar foods while you were low, this goes against what you are trying to do and only makes you feel much more unhappy. You will balance your blood sugar with Atkins, bring a jump in your step and stop the sugary 'highs' and 'lows.'

Cons:

The Atkins Diet admits that, in the initial phase of the program, dramatically reducing carbs will result in several side effects, such as:

- Headache
- Weakness
- Fatigue
- Constipation

- Weakness
- Dizziness

Also, carbs are so reduced by certain very low carb diets that they result in dietary shortages or inadequate fiber, which may cause health concerns such as nausea, diarrhea, and constipation.

However, consuming high-fiber, full-grain, and nutrient-dense carbohydrates will boost the nutritional profile of the Atkins Diet's initiatives. In comparison, to better avoid health issues, the Atkins Diet has evolved, and it now advises consuming a moderate quantity of additional sodium, along with nutrients or supplements.

It is also likely that ketosis can limit carbs to less than 20 grams a day, the amount prescribed for phase 1 of the diet. When you have not enough sugar (glucose) for power, ketosis happens because your body breaks down accumulated fat, allowing your body to build up ketones. Nausea, headache, emotional exhaustion, and foul breath can be side effects of ketosis.

Moreover, the Atkins Diet is not ideal for all. For starters, whether you are taking diuretics, oral diabetes or insulin drugs, the Atkins Diet advises that you contact a doctor before beginning the diet. Furthermore, individuals with serious kidney failure do not adopt the diet, and diet stages of weight reduction are not necessary for breastfeeding and pregnant people.

Some individuals who come to Atkins attempt their first diet, some have tried several various diets, but they have never found the best match. Anyway, we agree that the basic but powerful ideals of a low-carb lifestyle will help everyone.

In 2019, at both the American Society of Diet and the Diabetes Association conferences, announced findings from a broad nutritional analysis. The results show that there is not a particular diet that satisfies the needs of any person attempting to lose weight since each body reacts differently. These results reinforce studies reported in other scientific papers that show that the diet you will adhere to for the long-term is the safest diet for weight loss. And most diets for weight reduction, not just low-carb diets, can, at least momentarily, increase blood cholesterol or blood glucose levels. One research found that triglycerides were enhanced by persons who adopted the Atkins Diet, indicating improved cardiac protection. But no big studies have demonstrated whether those advantages hold on over the long run or improve how long you live.

6.2 Atkins vs. other Diet Programs:

There are lots of diets available today to choose from, and during your search to lose weight, you might have attempted quite a few. Here's how Atkins relates to other popular weight loss plans, plus more examples of why Atkins should be selected.

Over 80 scientific trials confirm the productivity and health effects of low-carb diets like Atkins. Research has found that low-carb diets like Atkins contribute to more successful weight loss and improved healthcare outcomes by comparing weight loss programs, such as a decline in heart failure and diabetes risk. Plus, to help you reduce weight and hold it off, Atkins can be adjusted to your particular needs.

Some examples below clarify why you can prefer Atkins diet plan over other diet plans:

Weight Watchers vs. Atkins Diet:

How it works:

Based on your current weight, gender, height, and age, you are assigned a regular calorie budget.

Things one must eat:

All foods are approved with a given number of points for each item (which equates to calories). Based on your regular calorie budget, you can consume the number of points.

Why Atkins diet is better:

Calorie-counting diets might not be successful since all calories are not treated the same way by your body. Your body is prompted to store fat with refined carbohydrates, added sugar and empty carbohydrates. Calorie-counting diets do not show you the food's nutritional importance or why specific food decisions can be taken, i.e., eliminating items that can contribute to weight gain. In other terms, you might waste the whole day's budget of points on Fries or candy on Weight Watchers, which are not nutritionally wise options that encourage weight loss. It is no match, Atkins vs. Weight Watchers!

Mediterranean vs. Atkins Diet

How it works:

Eat just like the Mediterranean culture.

Food one must take:

Many plant-based diets (fruits and veggies), rice, whole-grain wheat, grains, seeds, and nuts are safe to consume. Tiny amounts of milk, cheese, meat and eggs, shellfish and fish, and fats (not butter), and you can consume herbs and spices twice a week. Cut back on desserts and red meat.

Why Atkins diet is better:

When you are carbohydrate insensitive, this diet is difficult since you might be eating more carbohydrates than your body can manage. You will learn to understand your tolerance for carbohydrates on Atkins, which will help you lose weight and sustain it. You are often required to eat higher protein levels, which helps keep you happy during meals for longer.

Paleo vs. Atkins Diet

How it works:

Eat the same meal that the hunter-gatherer descendants and pre-agricultural consumed.

Food one must eat:

Grass-fed meats, seafood/fish, new fruits and veggies, nuts/seeds, eggs, and organic oils could be consumed. Cereal crops, legumes (such as peanuts), dairy, added sugar, carbohydrates, canned meats, highly oily foods, and processed vegetable oils, processed candy/junk/and fast foods should be avoided.

Why Atkins diet is better:

It insists on the quality but not the number of carbs (meaning you might overdo it), and with its concentration on grass-fed meats and sustainable ingredients, Paleo is more strict than Atkins. You can use processed foods on Atkins, like low-carb bars, drinks, and meals, making it simpler to stick to the Atkins diet, and that you are allowed to consume legumes and milk.

Keto vs. Atkins diet:

How it works:

The purpose of the keto diet is to push your body to use a certain fuel type. The keto diet plan depends on the ketone bodies, a form of fuel that the liver generates from stored fat, instead of depending on sugar (glucose) from carbohydrates (like beans, legumes, fruits, and vegetables).

Food one must take:

Green beans, asparagus, shellfish, fish, cheese, cabbage, avocado, broccoli, cauliflower, cucumber, meat, green beans, eggplant, kale, lettuce, olives, eggs, olive oil.

Why Atkins diet is better?

For those searching for a less restrictive, quite familiar plan, Atkins might be a better match. Besides certain minor side effects such as fatigue, nausea, irritability and poor breath, little short-term health effects are being recorded for Atkins. Keto can pose health hazards for people with some medical problems and is not deemed safe for liver or kidney conditions. Dramatic effects on reproductive hormones and insulin can involve hormonal changes. The use of keto for diabetes patients remains problematic, especially for those taking insulin.

Why Atkins low carb diet wins:

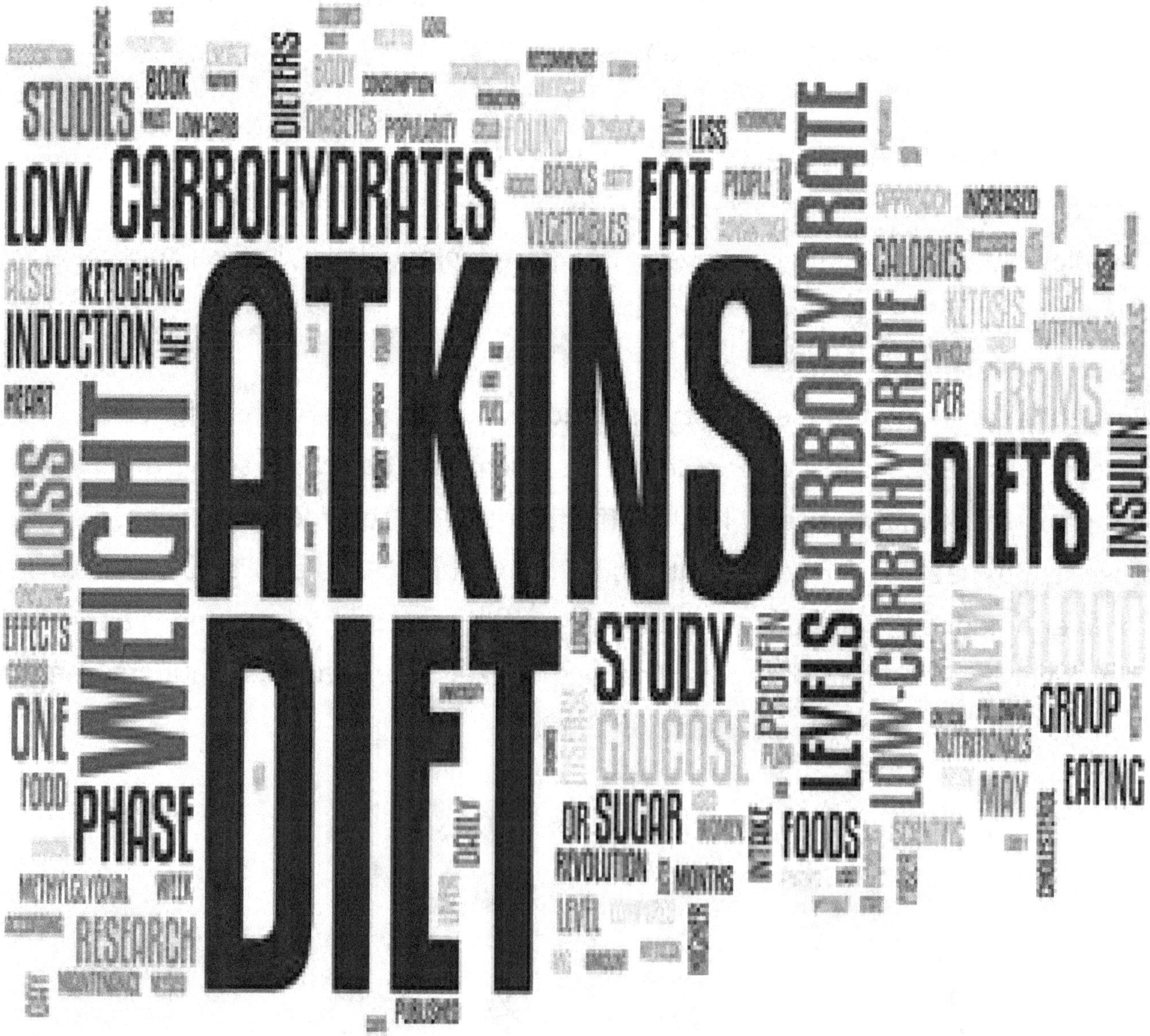

Atkins is a simple winner when analyzing diets. You will customize the proportions and kinds of carbs you can consume while also being able to reduce weight or sustain a fat loss, and you will think about the regulation of portions and the consistency of your diet and how your weight loss is influenced. kPlus Atkins is endorsed by over 80 research trials and offers various healthy low-carb choices that help make things much simpler to adhere to the diet, such as shakes, snacks and frozen meals.

6.3 Recent research:

For quite a few years, this diet has been around, but its popularity has grown in the past decade. Over the last few years, the Atkins Diet has been a popular subject globally, and there are several web resources and community groups accessible where dieters can get guidance about different food concerns.

The diet would undoubtedly continue to be a divisive topic for years to come, given its huge celebrity following and regular press exposure. Every dieter who has any reservations over implementing such a strict dietary schedule should

As low-carb diets have risen in popularity, a variety of experiments have been performed by researchers to determine the efficacy and additional health consequences of the diets. The Harvard School of Public Health states that some evidence suggests that low-carb diets will help individuals shed weight faster and manage it more than low-fat diets would, and that moderately low-carb diets could be heart-healthy as long as healthier foods come from protein and fat choices.

A previous meta-analysis looked at 23 randomized trials of more than 2,500 participants. The researchers noticed that participants on a low-fat diet observed a slight yet statistically important reduction in overall cholesterol and triglyceride levels relative to participants on a low-fat diet, and at least comparable declines in weight, waist size, and other disease risk details. Another research, reported in The BMJ in October 2018, showed that low-carb dieters were able to sustain weight loss because, relative to those on a diet of higher carbohydrates, they burned around 200 extra calories per day.

A famous nutritionist Popeck cautions said: "Cutting out carbohydrates will initially lead to weight loss. However, it is possibly wasteful and deficient in nutrients to remove whole food classes, such as grains, milk, yogurt, and berries " "Fiber will definitely be lacking, as well as potassium, calcium and other vitamins and minerals."

People interested in Atkins, but not consuming meat may opt to adopt the diet of Eco Atkins. The plan, established by researchers at Toronto's St. Michael's Hospital, has a comparable protein and carbohydrate ratio to the initial Atkins diet but substitutes vegetable protein with high-fat animal protein. For vegans and vegetarians, this diet is advisable. Customers that adopt a gluten-free lifestyle can have choices at Atkins. In addition to offering gluten-free meals, many gluten-free items are now sold by Atkins. Thus, the Atkins diet is the most well-known of the low-carb diets. The Atkins diet expects an extreme reduction in carbohydrates to less than 5 percent of the overall calorie consumption. The most contentious aspect of the Atkins plan is the simulated free-for-all consumption of as much protein and fat as you like.

Limiting sugary and starchy carbohydrates can help decrease calories and enable weight reduction for the individual who wants structure in their diet. And the safe and sensible thing to do is to rely onfats and proteins that are plant-based.

One must step away from the original Atkins 20 diet for your long-term wellbeing. It is the later stages of the diet that offer the range of foods that are necessary for health, particularly the Atkins 40. As you continue consuming almonds, peas, beans, vegetables and fruits, and whole grains again, and must work out and maintain portions small.

All of us try to cut out foods that we realize are terrible for us while trying to lose weight, be it fizzy beverages, indulgent sweets, or bread-based items. It is certain kinds of sugary, processed carbohydrates that will help you pack on weight. This makes common sense. You minimize the number of carbohydrates you consume with Atkins but take things much further: your body's metabolism switches to burning fat for energy. According to the firm, the items are not approved gluten-free by any third-party agency, but they fulfill the FDA's criteria.

The Atkins Plan, and others like it, went against the health recommendations and evidence that has been pushed out across the years: many nutritionists have been horrified by the prospect of a diet so high in fat and so poor in carbohydrates, and yet it has been shown to function. However, there are also questions among clinicians regarding the long-term effects that diets such as this can have.

Conclusion

While virtually thousands of fad diets are being marketed over the years, if we would not discuss the "Atkins Diet," the most popular mass diet of all times, we would be remiss. Robert Atkins created this high-protein, low-carbohydrate, high-fat diet. Dieters with allergies or hypersensitivity to grains, flour, and yeast could do quite well with this diet since carbohydrates are incredibly restricting and do not accommodate much in the way of bread or pasta, particularly during the initial crucial period.

However, eggs and fish, all of which are usually linked to food allergies, are key protein sources in this diet. Dieters should also make sure that they may not have an allergic reaction to foods like these before embarking on this plan. This would improve the diet's efficacy as well as decrease some health hazards. Try purchasing or lending one of the Atkins books if you are concerned about the Atkins diet, and please get started as soon as you can. Once of the followers of Atkins diet namely Shirley Hardy said:

"Atkins diet worked for me and there is no reason it cannot work for other people. I am 38 kg lighter now and the aching joints I suffered with when I was nearly 16 years old and it is a thing of the past. I have more energy and feel healthier than I have for a long time."

Ultimately, the safest diet for weight loss and other health issues is the one that a person practices to reach and sustain healthier body weight, so the Atkins diet is a strong and productive way to lose weight and stay healthy at the end of the day. You are not going to be disappointed.

Renal Diet Cookbook for beginners

The Best Beginners Cookbook With Easy And Delicious Recipes With Low Sodium and Low Potassium For Avoiding Dialysis

By

Maria Cox

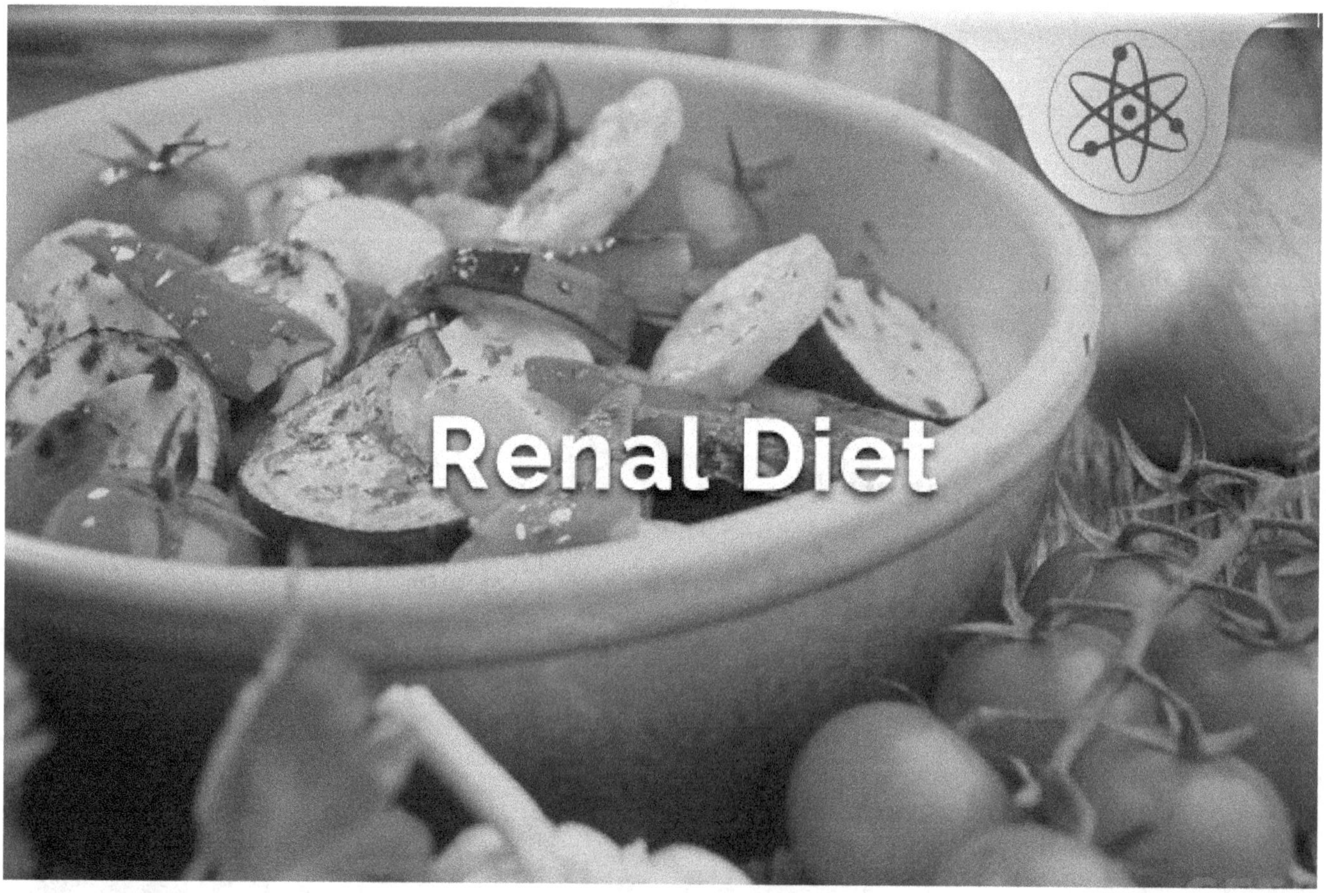
Renal Diet

Introduction

During recent history, kidney disease had become more prominent and widespread in the United States of America. The responsibility rests on us to know about the disease as much as we can. If somehow we catch this Chronic Kidney Disease (CKD), it is an education and knowledge that can empower us to fight against this harmful disease. The kidney is an essential organ in the human body, responsible for maintaining human health to keep it healthy and free of any misbalance inside the body. The kidney has several functions to execute, making it a vital and crucial human organ. Also, an increase in functions increases the risk of this organ, which needs to be addressed wisely within a suitable time.

On average, the size of the kidney is almost similar to that of the computer mouse. The Kidney's basic functions inside our body include cleaning and filtering blood, producing red blood cells, and removing waste or toxic substances absorbed in the blood.

Basic Kidney Functions

The kidney is a small organ, but it can do some powerful functions in our body. Their shape is like that of a bean, and their size is almost equal to a hand fist or the mouse of a computer. It is located slightly below the rib cage. When it is in a perfect state, Kidneys carry out some important functions like:

- Managing the blood pressure through releasing hormones that control variation in blood pressure
- Making blood free of any waste product through filtration
- Helping in production of red blood cells through stimulation of bone marrow that makes red blood cells
- Removing extra water or any fluid present inside the human body
- Strengthening of bones through the production of vitamin D

Chapter 1: Kidney Disease and its Types

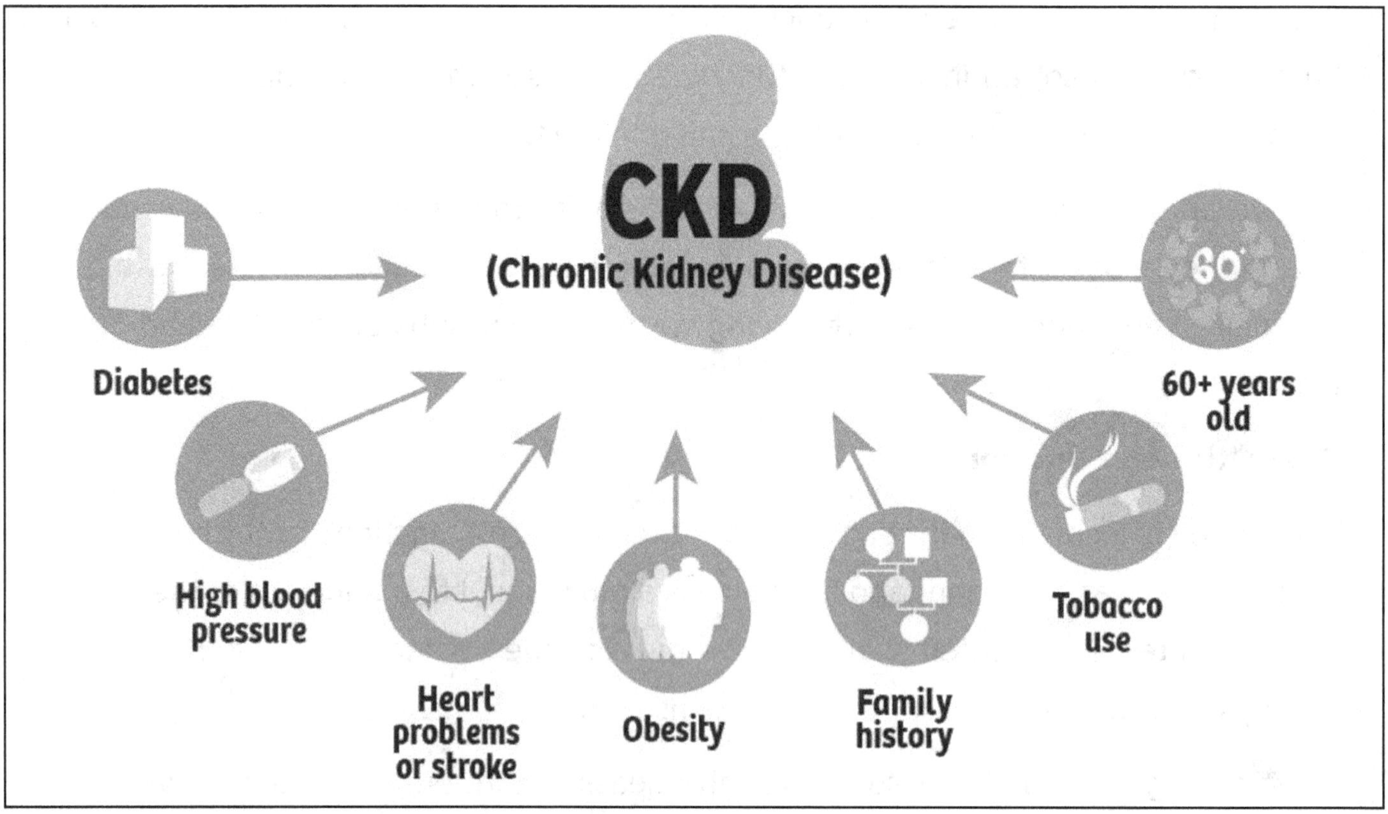

1.1. Sources of Kidney disease

There is no specific single cause of kidney disease. Kidney disease can be caused by a physical injury that can damage the kidney along with other organs. According to data collected by doctors, although there is no single reason that can only be announced as the cause of kidney disease, there are two prominent causes common in kidney disease patients: high blood pressure and diabetes. Diagnosing this disease at the initial stage and striving to contain it from day one can slow down its progression to help you get rid of the disease and prevent you from a heart attack and stroke.

When protein is digested in our body, some waste is produced. These waste products move to the urine when blood is circulated into our capillaries. Blood accumulate red blood cells and proteins because, due to their size, they are unable to move inside our veins, sometimes called capillaries. All the filtration of blood is done by the kidney hence taking the toll on waste products. But when the kidney gets damaged, it starts malfunctioning, allowing some of the waste to move along the blood into our capillaries, affecting several other organs. If the disease is diagnosed at early stages, it is more likely to get controlled through several known treatments. However, suppose it is not diagnosed timely. In that case, it can lead to the accumulation of high protein in patient urine, known as microalbuminuria, resulting in end-stage renal disease.

Secondly, hypertension, another term for high blood pressure, is also the most common cause of kidney disease. Hypertension can only be controlled through certain medications and adopting a renal diet that lacks sodium contents. Daily exercise can also help to control blood pressure. Under normal conditions, Kidneys manage the blood pressure inside the body. Still, when a person suffers from high blood pressure, it overburdens his heart that needs to exert extra power to pump the blood into capillaries. In contrast, the capillaries get stretched when subjected to the high pressure of blood to let the maximum amount of blood pass through them that causes the capillaries or blood vessels all over the body, including kidney's blood vessel to promote malfunctioning of different organs. Kidneys cannot remove waste products from the blood with injured blood vessels, resulting in a difficult blood circulation cycle inside the patient's body.

Those people having diabetes suffers from high blood sugar in their bloodstreams. Thus blood containing high sugar contents can deplete blood vessel walls and the kidney walls and contribute to high blood pressure. Furthermore, it can be claimed that diabetes can be a cause of high blood pressure, and it can foster chances of a heart attack.

Thirdly, the auto-immune disease can be a source of kidney disease. The auto-immune disease involves the functioning of the immune system, which protects the human body in case of illness- against the body's benefit. In this disease, the immune system considers the human body as its enemy and triggers its resources to defeat a person's system. In addition to that, good pasture, the syndrome, can be a kidney failure source. It is also a kind of an autoimmune disease. These autoimmune diseases are so critical that they can lead to kidney failure from where there is no come back except kidney transplant.

1.2. Chronic Kidney Disease Treatment plan

To deal with this kind of difficult disease, a strong determination is needed. The patient must consciously participate in clinical activities. Cooperation with the clinical team that is to assist a patient in countering that disease is very important. Apart from that, one must religiously and cautiously follow a well-planned renal diet and make some time for healthy activities like sports or walking.

Cooperation with the healthcare team

Cooperation with the healthcare team is the most important thing that a patient needs to keep in mind. It will help him improve his health condition, but it will keep them stick to their goal to fight against the disease without losing hope. Healthcare team members are always trained to trigger a motivating force among their patients to help patients in their speedy recovery. In addition to that, discussing with healthcare team members will allow patients to take suitable and firm decisions about their health and adopt their new lifestyle to improve their health.

Renal diet

The main focus in this book is on the renal diet. A renal diet is very important for those patients who are serious about tackling this disease. A renal diet can create a difference and change your health condition in no time, but the requirement is to follow it religiously and honestly. In the beginning, one can understand that it is difficult to adopt this diet because it demands a patient to stop consuming salt, cut down protein and consume a specific amount of calories, which is not an easy task for any person. Switching to a renal diet from a normal diet takes time, but this time can be shortened through the patient determination to cull this disease and the type of recipe he will select. Several alternatives to minerals like protein and salt can still keep the meal joyous for a patient. Still, if the patient is unaware of these ingredients, he has to eat meals with completely different tastes, making it difficult for them to adopt.

Healthy Lifestyle

A decision for a healthy lifestyle can result in a fruitful outcome. Introducing activities like sports, running, walking, or making out leisure time for oneself can positively impact mental and physical health. High blood pressure can also be caused by excessive stress and tension, while these activities can evade this cause, contributing to health amelioration.

1.3. Kinds of Kidney Failure

Initially, in normal practice, doctors use to observe the proliferation of creatinine levels in the blood. Once they suspect the increased creatinine level in the blood, they then know about the kind of kidney failure, whether it is acute superimposed over chronic, acute, or chronic level. A simple description of these kinds is as following

- Acute superimposed over chronic causes immense damage to renal function of a patient suffering from kidney failure.
- Chronic is a condition that continues for a long period
- Acute is a condition or suffering that is very intense and painful but never lasts long.

After knowing the kidney disease, the doctors' next step is to map out the duration of kidney failure. It is difficult to map out the duration, so the first pinpoint the main cause of kidney failure because it can happen for several reasons. Once doctors can know the cause of failure, they use it to determine the duration of kidney failure.

Urine and blood testing is the most reliable source for doctors to know the presence and cause of kidney failure. Urinalysis is a process in which doctors use to conduct urine tests in which they use to note down the presence of minerals like Phosphate, calcium, electrolytes, creatinine, and urea nitrogen. In blood tests, they use to count the presence of red blood cells because those patients who suffer from kidney failure undergo plummeting red blood cell production. Elevated creatinine and the abnormal urinalysis history can be used as a vital tool for differentiation between acute kidney disease from chronic kidney disease.

In some cases, the renal functions use to decline to such an extent that they reach end-stage kidney disease. In such circumstances, it becomes difficult for doctors to carry out an accurate diagnosis. For patients who reach this stage, doctors use a kidney biopsy to make a precise diagnosis. Also, there are conditions for carrying out a biopsy; there must not be a small excessive fiber tissue present; otherwise, the biopsy disadvantages will top up biopsy advantages. To know whether the conditions are suitable or not, doctors use to observe the ultrasound reports before going for the biopsy to know whether the benefits of biopsy will outweigh its disadvantages or not.

1.4. Treatment for kidney patients

Patients who are diagnosed with kidney failure have to choose between two options. If they have the resources to look for a kidney donor, they can go for it, and it is the best option; otherwise, they have to go for dialysis.

Dialysis is a process in which artificial means are used to eliminate extra fluid and toxins that get accumulated inside a patient's kidney. It is an expensive process, and it has to be carried at short intervals again and again. Thus repeatedly carrying out this process makes it more uncomfortable and expensive.

On the other hand, kidney transplant is also an expensive process nut it has to be done once, making it a preferable choice. However, whatever the choice you make, there are several examples in the practical world that patients who had chosen either option live a healthy life. It does not matter whether you chose dialysis over a kidney transplant or vice versa. It is advised not to lose hope and remain positive with whatever resources you have.

1.5. Types of Dialysis

Hemodialysis

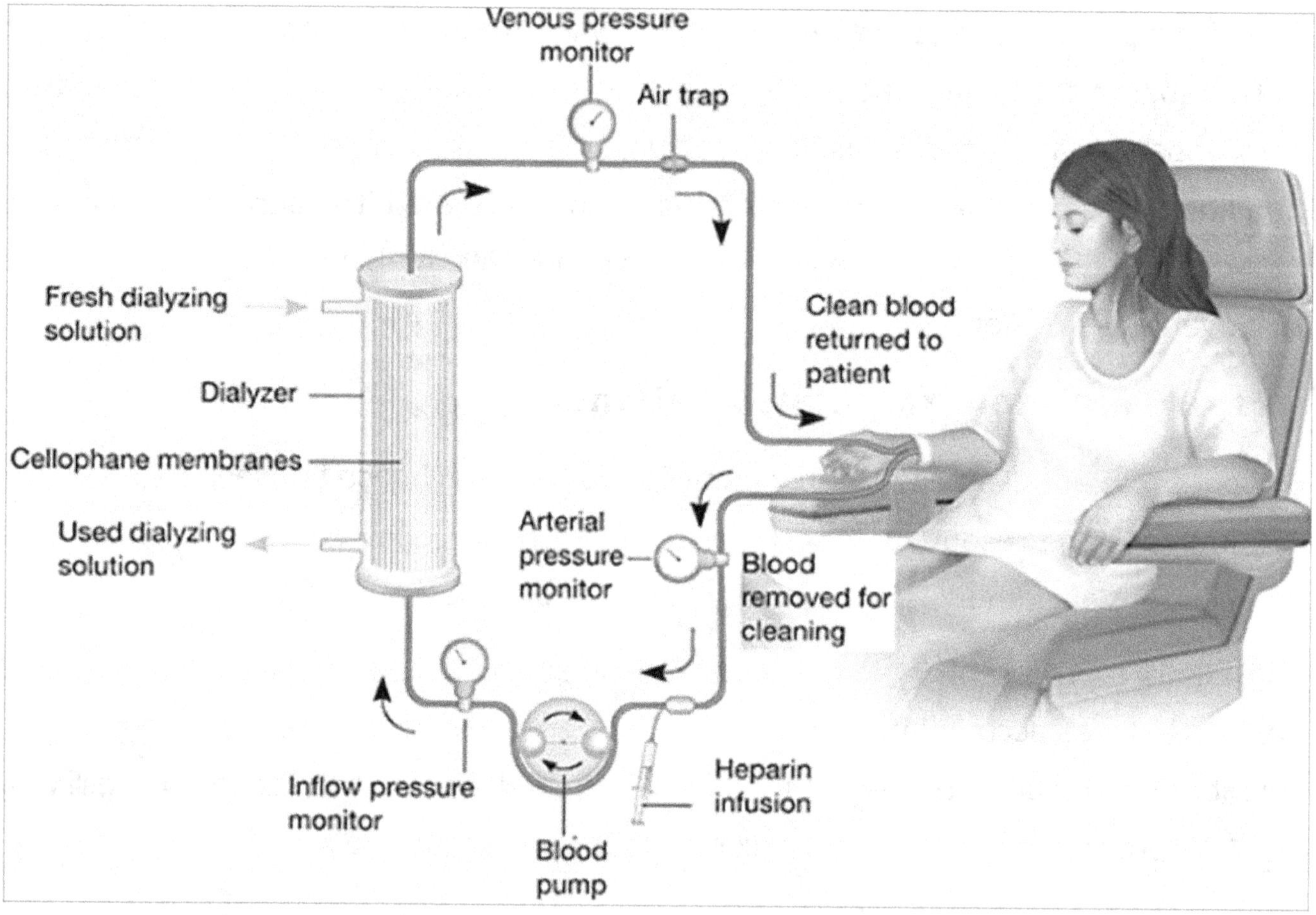

hemodialysis is also called 'hemo.' This type of dialysis is most commonly carried out in the case of kidney failure. Hemodialysis involves the use of a special kind of machine to filter out and clean patient blood. This process can be carried out at home, but it is preferred to perform at the hospital or clinic if the patient's budget allows him.

Peritoneal Dialysis

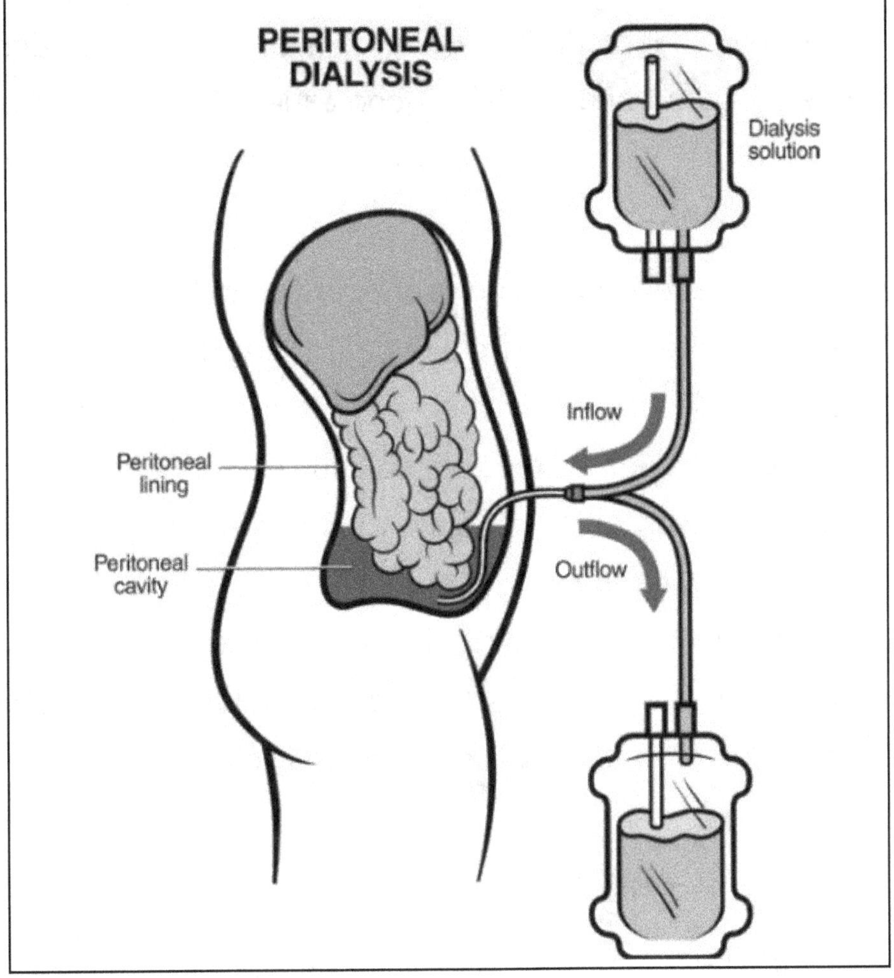

This process involves lining the patient's abdominal area and a Dialysate solution to clean the patient's blood. The interesting fact about this technique is that it can be carried out at home until and unless provided the surrounding area is clean.

Kidney Transplant

As the name suggests, a kidney transplant includes surgery in which a healthy kidney of a donor replaces the patient's failed kidney. An alive donor can donate the new kidney, or a dead person can donate it for a good cause. Aside from that, there is another alternative, but it does not present any reliable permanent solution. That alternate is medical management.

Medical management is suitable for those who cannot afford those highly expensive solutions to their disease. This alternate will help mitigate the intensity of symptoms, and your kidney will keep working until it completely fades away and gets broke down. If a patient intends to choose that medical solution, it is important for him to consult any wise physician who can guide him in a much better way. The physician will help draw a suitable plan indicating all the dos and what the patient should not do. Medical management also includes hospice care. In hospice care, the main focus is to reduce the patient's pain and make his last days as comfortable as possible. Most patients who cannot avail of those expensive options select the hospice for the rest of their life.

In hospice, the patient can expect the following things:

- Hospice will help patient's relatives and close one to support the patient morally and mentally
- Hospice will provide a proper medication plan to keep the patient's pain to a minimal level and will help follow the medication plan thoroughly
- Hospice can provide a nurse to take care of patient 24/7
- Hospice will surely help improve the quality remaining life of a patient.

In the beginning, the patient has to face problems to adjust himself to a new routine, but with the passage, the routine becomes a habit, and then the patient starts enjoying it wholeheartedly. The patient will start enjoying the company of Nurses, their relatives, loved ones, neighboring patients, and everyone else.

Chapter 2: How to manage kidney disease

2.1. Stress handling while being a Kidney patient

It is quite an important subject for those suffering from lethal kidney failure because stress is directly linked with one of the major causes of this disease. Stress contributes to high blood pressure, which affects the already damaged kidney system, leading to more pain and worsening health. Patients need to understand that life is full of hurdles, and every hurdle brings along a multitude of stress with it, and it is them who need to handle it to pull their life out of greater risk. Following are some of the tips that can help any kidney patient to keep stress at bay:

- Always make out some time to relax your mind and body. I prefer meditation, deep breathing, and visualization.
- Include exercise in your timetable. This will help you manage stress and provide an environment to think out of the box and feel more relax.
- When the patient feels that he is under intense stress, he must prefer calling his best friend or loved one to divert his attention and motivation.
- Always think constructively. The patient must not try to change what is not under his control. Using your power against unconquerable is sheer foolishness that will bring nothing except the loss of power and gain of misery.
- To keep the depression at the door, the patient must not keep any expectations from anyone.
- Everyone is prone to making mistakes, so when a patient makes any mistake, he must not take it to his heart and just let it go to avoid any further loss.

Apart from adopting a renal diet, physicians suggest another way of keeping good health and improving lifestyle. Exercise is a much better option; it will not help you maintain your health but will put new colors in a patient's life. In the beginning, one can understand that it is quite difficult to do daily exercise, especially when the patient intends to do it alone. Still, once the momentum is developed, it will surely drag the patient towards his destination without demanding much input. If a perfect exercise schedule accompanies a renal diet, it would be a perfect combination. The patient will indirectly be getting more benefits from this combination than he must have expected; it will help him reduce weight, remain physically fit, deep and serene sleep, muscles building and feeling full of energy all the time, and many more.

Furthermore, a study has shown that those who walk up to 10,000 steps daily and work almost two and a half-hour daily and cutting down 500-800 calories daily, and thoroughly follow their balanced diet plan have around about 50 percent chance of mitigating blood sugar level in their body which surely assists them in achieving good health and a healthy lifestyle.

The good thing for patients interested in including daily exercise in their routine is that several options are available about different exercise types. Each exercise is as beneficial as the other one. From several exercises, the patient will find it easy to develop his interest in at least one of them. The joy of this exercise will keep him motivated to keep sticking to the routine. Following are the most common and most effective exercise that physician highly recommends to their patients to adopt:

- Stretching
- Running
- Swimming
- Gamming (that may include any physical game like any kind of sport)
- Swimming
- Cycling
- Yoga

- Boating
- Hiking
- Stair Climbing

There is no need to take a membership to perform all these exercises. Even the patient is not required to buy any expensive gadget for it. All these exercises aim to maintain health that can also be achieved by buying a simple walk around the street and performing a brief yoga at home.

Protein Intake Restriction

Protein is the major source of maintenance and restoration of tissues inside our body. It is a protein that helps fight against germs and infection whenever there is an internal or external injury. However, it is recommended to those patients who are not having a dialysis treatment yet must avoid an excess of protein to reduce the renal function rate. This will also contribute to delaying the requirement of dialysis and transplantation of renal. It must be noted that protein is not cut down to zero value because if it happens, it can lead to malnutrition and patient weakness. An intense restriction on protein consumption, improper diet, fatigue, and body resistance loss contributes to death chances of kidney disease patients. High protein like meat, fish, eggs, poultry, and alike must be consumed to balance. But patients having chronic kidney disease are advised to restrain from consuming such high protein items. Similarly, those working on their muscle growth must avoid consuming creatinine substances because it can put patients' lives in danger.

Fluid intake

One of the kidney's main functions is to remove the water or any other fluid from the body in the form of urea. In patients suffering from chronic kidney disease, the amount of urea plummets due to the kidney's malfunction. The decrease in urea means that the blood's waste will go unfiltered and the blood into the veins. This waste can cause swelling of hands and legs, swelling of veins, and swelling of different body organs. It also contributes to high blood pressure. Accumulation of fluid inside the lungs can be dangerous, resulting in the shortening of breath. It can cost a life if it is ignored for a long time.

There is a misconception that patients suffering from kidney disease must take a large quantity of fluid daily to keep their kidneys healthy. The amount of consumption of water depends upon the condition of the patient's kidney. Water intake should be contained to a required level because it can promote further swelling. To reduce swelling, it is advised that the patient must intake fluid lesser than the volume of urine produced. Patients diagnosed with edema must increase water intake by 500 ml each day to compensate for the loss of fluid by exhalation and perspiration.

Keeping the record of the Patient's weight

To keep an eye on the quantity of fluid gained or lost by the patient, it is important to keep the patient weight daylight. It is important to maintain the body's weight, and it can only happen if the patient religiously follows all the assigned instructions to him by his physician. An increase in the weight of the patient can be dangerous. An increase in weight means an increase in water volume or fluid inside the body, which means the patient needs to impose more intense fluid intake restrictions. On the flip side, weight reduction can also be dangerous too because it can lead to weak health, and it is an indicator that the imposed restriction is more than the required level.

There are several ways to reduce the amount of water intake. The patient must be careful in consuming substances that increase thirsts like fish, salt, or spices. Likewise, patients must not drink water as a habit or because someone else drinks it too much, so what shall he do. Using small cups of water can also help in reducing fluid consumption. Patients who have diabetes feel more thrust due to high blood sugar levels in their body, so it is required to keep the blood sugar to its suitable level by abstaining from carrying out such activities, resulting in increased blood sugar levels.

A most common and widespread kind of kidney disease is chronic kidney disease

2.2. Chronic Kidney Disease(CKD)

To prevent any disease, it is important to know about the basics of that disease. CKD (Chronic Kidney Disease) is a disease about the malfunction of the Kidney. It is usually caused by high blood pressure and diabetes. According to the observation gathered from different health clinics of the United States, it has been revealed that every 1 out of every three persons having diabetes or high blood pressure suffers from CKD. When a person suffers from Chronic Kidney Disease (CKD), it causes toxic and unfiltered blood containing different undesirable and unfavorable chemicals and wastes to circulate to different parts of our body, rendering a decrease in their efficiency.

The most dangerous thing about CKD (Chronic Kidney Disease) is that its symptoms are not conspicuous, which helps this disease advance and take a stronger position inside the human body, causing more damage to different body organs. It is important to pinpoint this disease while in the initial phase before it grows its roots deep to prevent excessive damage. Initially, the disease does not show any prominent symptoms that lead most people to ignore this evil. Still, when it gets to advance an alarming level, people decide to get their body check against that disease. This disease can be diagnosed through two available means of testing: Urine tests and blood samples. The Urine test involves measuring the protein contents in the urine. Simultaneously, in blood samples, testing includes measuring or detecting creatinine, a waste product usually found in the blood when the Kidney undergoes malfunctioning. Besides these procedures, there are some other alternatives, e.g., knowing Kidney numbers like Estimated glomerular filtration rate

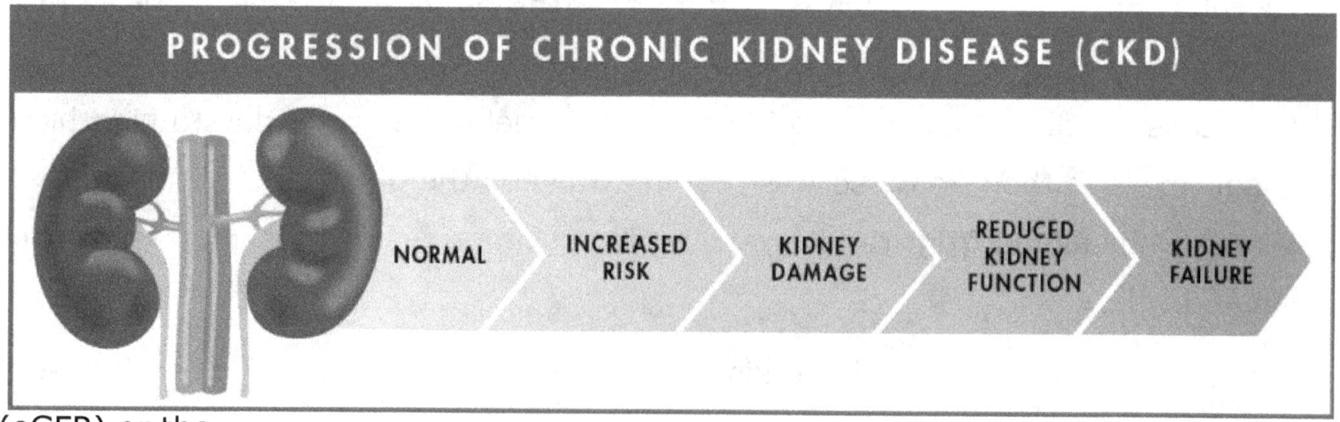

(eGFR) or the

extent of albumin, a protein, slippage in the urine.

The kidney number that you must know:

- The estimated glomerular filtration rate (eGFR) shows the rate of blood filtered by our kidney per minute.
- Whereas in alternate method quantity of albumin is measured in urine because albumin is a protein that gets through the Kidney as a waste into the urine when the Kidney is damaged and undergoing malfunctioning.

Symptoms of CKD

- Itching
- Vomiting and Nausea
- Feet and ankle swelling
- Muscle cramps
- Feeling trouble in breathing
- Unable to Sleep or feeling trouble in doing so
- Loss of hunger
- Having not enough Urine or having an excess of Urine.

Consequences of CKD (Chronic Kidney Disease)

Some of the prominent consequences of CKD include:

- CKD can result in loss or lack of red blood cells or Anemia
- An increase in the level of phosphorous and potassium and plummeting of the level of calcium such growing is adverse for human health
- Increase in probability of catching infection inside the body due to circulation of unclean and unfiltered blood
- Worsening in quality of life through the development of overwhelming depression
- Weakness due to loss of hunger or appetite to eat

Chapter 3: The Meal Plan for Kidney Patients

This book discussion would be based on how to evade and get rid of this unwelcome disease. If you are fearful of catching this disease or doubtful about its presence inside your body or already a victim of this disease, I am sure that you have got your hands on the right book. To keep this kind of disease at bay or contain its progression, it is important to remain conscious of your diet plan. Our main focus would be on a suitable diet plan for kidney patients and those who want to protect themselves from this disease.

For kidney patients, renal diet is of prime focus. In the early 20th century, this diet was recommended by scientists after observing its benefits for a kidney. Since then, thousands of people suffering from Kidney disease have improved their health and have kept kidney disease at bay.

A renal diet's basic concept is to control your consumption of sodium, phosphorous, potassium, and protein. It has been observed that consumption of a calculated amount of these minerals can help prevent and recover for Kidney disease.

Phosphate

Usually, under normal circumstances, phosphate consumption is not dangerous, but kidney patient care needs to be taken while consuming phosphate. It is direly perilous to consume phosphate when your kidney is damaged up to 80 percent. It is advised to consider the decrease in phosphate intake by counting the consumption of calories and minerals.

Potassium

Once diagnosed that the patient is running high on Potassium intake, it is advised to decrease potassium consumption as an excess of everything is dangerous. Baked potatoes are a vital potassium source, while leafy green juices of fruits also have high potassium contents, which need to be cut down from the patient diet. However, the number of other fruit items and vegetables containing little or no potassium contents can be joyfully consumed.

Sodium

It is a main salt and salt component and one of the most commonly used items in our dishes. But when you are suffering from kidney disease, you have to restrain from consuming sodium in any form. Although it is a difficult task, it needs to be done to maintain your health. As quoted above, high blood pressure can be the cause of Chronic Kidney disease(CKD), and sodium conduces to high blood pressure, so that is why it must be cut from your diet otherwis3e to be a harmful content for kidney patient health. However, if sodium is cut down from the patient's diet, it does not mean that he cannot enjoy tasty meals anymore. Still, there are several alternatives to sodium that needs to be searched that can help give a patient's diet a joyous taste. That search is made easy by us in this book—the attendant needs to select one of the recipes in this book and cook food following quoted instructions. Herbs and spices can be a good alternative. Use of mustard, garlic, or pepper can replace salt by imparting your food a similar taste to sodium salt.

Recipes quoted in this book are some of the simplest, easiest, and clearly defined recipes. All these recipes are also healthy too. This book is helpful for beginners and for those who are already used to following a renal diet. Beginners will surely find it easy and surprisingly joyous, while those who had already adopted a renal diet can use this book to impart a new taste to their diet.

The renal diet proposed in this book is a sodium-free diet. Usually, the alternatives to sodium that most people use to select are potassium or fiber and content having low sodium. However, most people find it difficult and confusing to increase the fiber intake because, in the usual diet, they consider excess fiber consumption unhealthy. Still in renal diet

3.1. Buying CKD friendly staples

It is a wise choice always to plan that will help save time and achieve more comfort. Here are some of the tips patient must consider while selecting CKD friendly staples from a grocery shop

It is important to read the label on every product, especially those who have any disease and follow a specific diet plan. CKD patients must consider the amount of sodium quoted on the nutrition fact list long with potassium in food items they will buy.

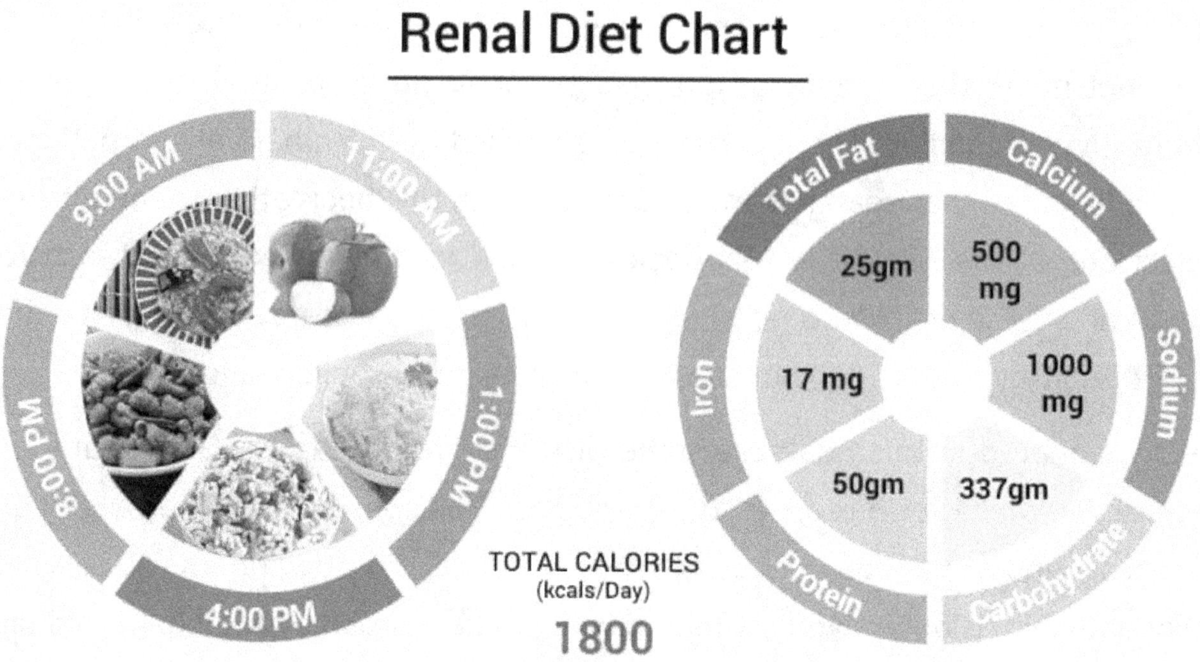

Consider those products o food items containing a minimal amount of sodium or salt contents in it. It sometimes happens that the patient gets fed up with the taste of old food, and he wanted to change the taste, but unluckily he does not find any salt free food item to cook. In this situation, rinse that food item thoroughly before cooking it and prefer consuming frozen vegetables.

For protein intake, the best option is bean consumption. But suppose the patient is confronting a severe level of chronic kidney disease. In that case, his physician might be advised to count on phosphorous and potassium consumption, and consuming beans is not an appreciable choice.

The preparation of dried beans personally is a great idea. It will help reduce the amount of sodium in these dried beans, making the beans cheap and healthy for the patient. But if the patient prefers the canned beans, it is important to rinse these beans thoroughly before they are set for cooking.

Always prefer to purchase those canned fruits that are packed in water

- The same approach must be kept in mind while buying canned fish or chicken.
- Always go for the salt-free version of snacks that the patient like to eat
- It is pertinent to consider the expiry date of all the food items the patient will buy.

3.2. Basics of a healthy diet

There are four basic nutrients that everyone who follows any diet plan needs to consider on the nutrition list of any food item they will buy from the grocery shop. These nutrients are as following

- Fat
- Calories
- Carbohydrates
- Protein

The main purpose of providing a nutrition fact list on each food item is to help consumers keep balance in their diet plan by considering that list. Now let us discuss these four basic nutrients briefly.

Fats

Everyone needs some quantity of fat in their meal to keep themselves healthy. Fat imparts energy to the human body and helps extract energy from vitamins present in the food items. The major problem caused by overconsumption of fat is the increase in weight loss. Apart from this, it can also lead to heart disease if its consumption is not timely controlled. Among the different types of fats, unsaturated fats are considered as the healthier or good fats. Olive oil, corn oil, and peanut oil are the major source of unsaturated fats.

Cholesterol levels can be controlled through the consumption of unsaturated fats. Those who are intended to increase their weight can achieve their goal through excessive intake of unsaturated fats

On the other hand, there are saturated fats too that are severely dangerous for health. Saturated fats raise the cholesterol level that increases the risk of heart disease. Meats, lard, butter, and shortening are some of the sources of saturated fats.

Calories

Calories are also the source of energy for a body. Fat, protein, and carbohydrates are the main source of calories. The number of calories required by the human body depends upon the age of a person. In addition to that, sometimes people need to adjust the number of calories to gain or lose weight.

Carbohydrates

Carbs or carbohydrates are also a source of energy. Vegetables and fruits are the main sources of carbohydrates. Patients suffering from chronic kidney disease must consider consuming carbohydrates because they contain phosphorous and potassium. Kidney patients need to keep a strict count on these minerals. It is also important to consider carbohydrates because they also contribute to diabetes, and they also impact the blood sugar level.

Protein

Protein is called the building block of a body. Protein is a source of growth for the body. Lack of protein can result in different diseases like nail weakness, worsening skin, and hair fall. To remain healthy, it is important to keep a perfect balance in protein consumption. Usually, patients with kidney diseases are advised to restrict the protein intake because malfunctioning of the kidney never lets the protein be handled properly, hence overburdening the kidney, leading to further harm to the organ. Based on the quantity of protein present in the food item, a following lower and higher protein classification is done by nutritionists. Pasta, rice, fruits, bread, and vegetables are categorized as low protein food items, while fish, red meat, eggs, and poultry are set in a high protein category.

Sodium

It is also important to consider the sodium contents list on each food item's nutrition fact list along with those four basic nutritional items. Salt is a mineral found in every food item, and kidney patients are strictly barred from consuming an excess of salt. Salt causes an increase in blood pressure hence putting hard kidney heart at greater risk.

""""*

3.3. Kidney friendly Lifestyle

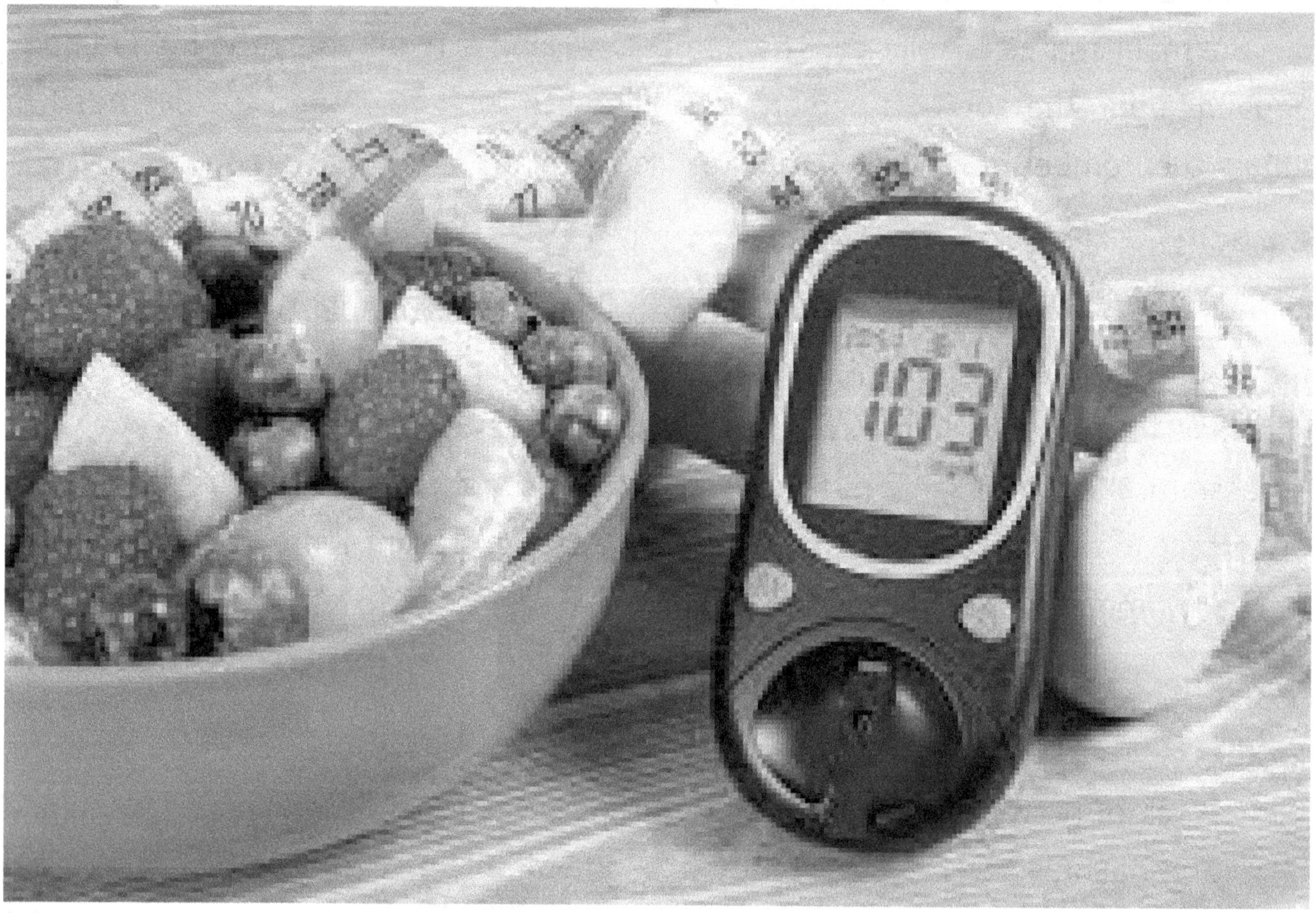

Whenever any patient is diagnosed with Kidney disease, the first and foremost tool they look for to counter and restrict the expansion of the disease is a balanced and healthy diet that would help control blood pressure and blood sugar; as mentioned earlier that it is not easy to adopt renal diet so easy and leave your previous joyous diet. Still, it is recommended that a patient adopt the following instructions to feel healthy and happy.

- Try to eat different kinds of food to help patients select different joyous foods when fed up with normal dishes. Exploring within renal diet constraints will surely help patients regain their joy while switching to a new diet.
- Happiness comes from your inside rather than from the outside world. Always try to enjoy whatever the meal is. It takes time to develop taste, but this patient has to give food a chance to develop his taste for a while.

- Try to minimize consumption of sodium as much as it is possible because it can ruin your whole internal system once you are diagnosed with kidney disease
- Before taking any multivitamin or any other supplement, consult your doctor or your health care team.
- Once you are diagnosed with kidney disease, keep following your physician's renal diet and avoid switching the diet on your own.

3.4. Slowing down and countering kidney disease

Even if you can keep your kidney working at the least possible working stage, it can still help you a lot. By protecting your kidney, you can save your heart and other organs from injury too. Following are the basic things that can be considered to avoid kidney failure:

- Kidney patients are more prone to the variation in blood sugar, and it can cost kidney failure and heart disease. High sugar contents may lead to swelling of blood vessels imparting immense damage to their walls. It is advised that if you are a victim of kidney disease, you must check your blood sugar variation before and after the meal to know the effects of the meal over blood sugar level inside your body. Cut back all those constituents from your meal that causes a rise in your blood sugar.
- A recent CARDIA study has revealed that those having extra weight are more prone to catch kidney disease than kidney disease. So, it has been advised that if you are overweight, try reducing your weight as much as you can.
- Smoking and other drugs are quite harmful to the kidney. The patient must quit such activities that can cost them their life.
- Blood pressure is an important factor that a patient must give a prime focus. An increase in blood pressure can be as harmful as a rise in blood sugar level. Always take medicine on time to maintain balanced blood pressure.

- Cut back protein from your diet as much as you can. Try to consume protein only to a moderate level; otherwise, it will have excess urea upon breaking down. As urea is hard to remove for already a damaged kidney, excess urea will demand more power from the kidney hence rendering it more prone to damage.

Chapter4:

Breakfast Recipes

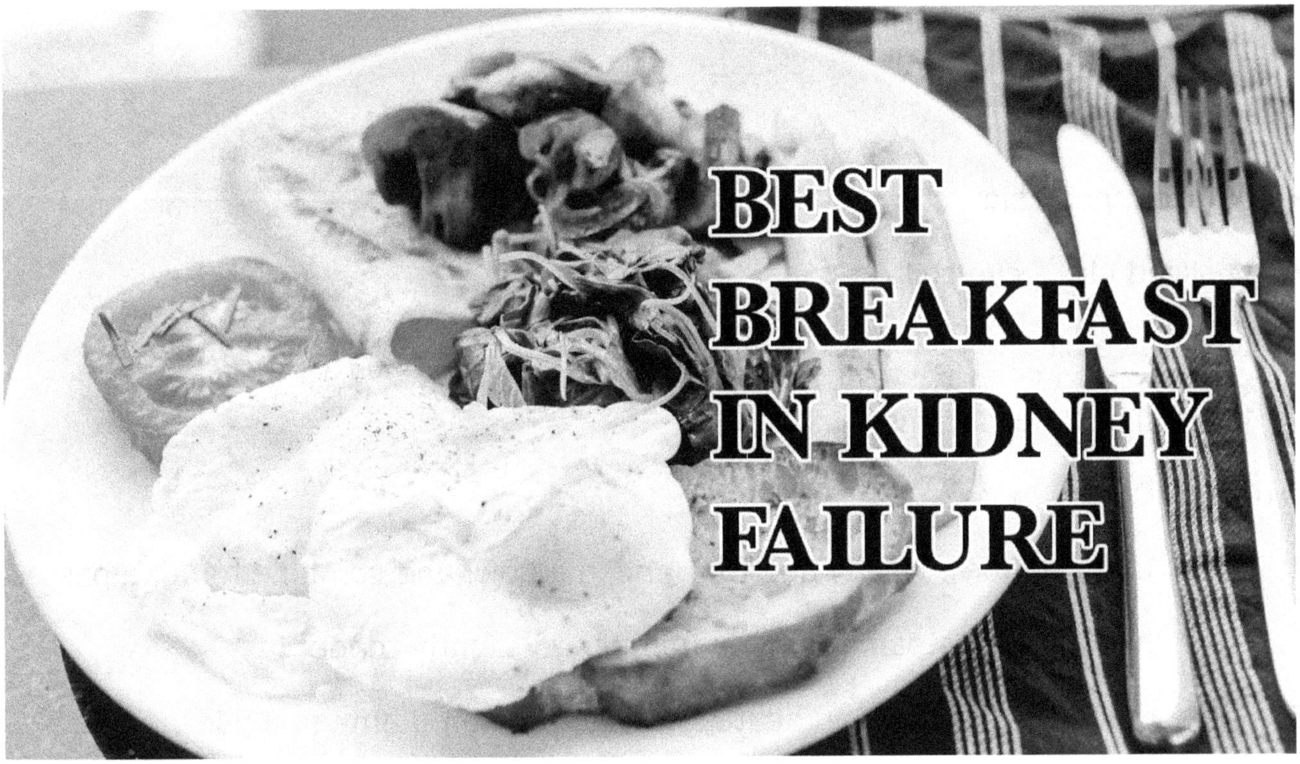

4.1. Sirtfood Mushrooms Scrambled Eggs

Ready in: 18 minutes

Servings: 3

Difficulty: Easy

INGREDIENTS

- ½ cup chopped parsley
- Two eggs
- 1 tsp curry powder, mild
- 1 tsp turmeric
- 20g chopped kale
- ½ sliced bird's eye chili
- 1 tsp olive oil
- 1 cup sliced mushrooms

DIRECTIONS

1. Whisk curry powder, water, and turmeric in a bowl and combine to get a paste.
2. Place the kale over steam for three minutes to slightly tender it.
3. Sauté mushroom and chili in heated oil over medium flame in a pan.
4. Mix in egg and cook for a minute.
5. Stir in curry paste and toss well.
6. Add kale and cook for two more minutes.
7. Transfer the mixture to the serving dish and add parsley. Toss well.
8. Serve and enjoy it.

NUTRITION: Calories: 557 kcal Fat: 21 g Protein: 11 g Carbs: 72 g

4.2. Sweet Potato Hash

Ready in: 30 minutes

Servings: 4

Difficulty: Medium

INGREDIENTS

- Two chopped garlic cloves
- 2 tbsp olive oil
- ½ diced white onion
- Three diced sweet potatoes, peeled
- Two chopped celery stalks
- ½ tsp black pepper
- 1 ½ tsp salt
- 1/3 cup chopped green onions for garnishing

DIRECTIONS

1. Sauté potatoes, celery, and onions in heated oil over medium flame in skillet.
2. Drizzle pepper and salt and toss well.
3. Cover the skillet and let it cook for 20 minutes with occasional stirring.
4. After 20 minutes, increase the flame and stir in garlic and toss well.
5. Cook for five more minutes.
6. Transfer the mixture to the serving dish.
7. Serve with onions and enjoy it.

NUTRITION: Calories: 157 cal Fat: 7 g Protein: 1 g Carbs: 22 g

4.3. Crunchy and Chewy Granola

Ready in: 80 minutes

Servings: 12

Difficulty: Medium

INGREDIENTS

- 2 cups mixed diced dried fruits
- ¼ cup honey
- Two egg whites
- ¼ cup maple syrup
- 1/3 cup vegetable oil
- 1 tsp cinnamon
- 1 tsp vanilla extract
- 1 tsp salt
- 4 cups oats
- ½ tsp orange zest, grated
- 1 cup diced nuts (any of your choice)

DIRECTIONS

1. Whisk egg whites, salt, honey, cinnamon, oil, orange zest, maple syrup, salt, and vanilla in a bowl.
2. Take half of the cup of batter out of the mixture in a separate bowl and mix in dried fruit in it. Keep the bowl aside for a while.
3. Stir in nuts and oats in the remaining mixture and whisk well to combine everything nicely.
4. Transfer the oat batter to a baking tray lined with butter paper.
5. Bake in a preheated oven at 275 Fahrenheit for 30 minutes.

6. Now mix in fruit mixture with oat mixture and spread an even layer of granola in a baking tray.
7. Bake for 40 minutes in a preheated oven at 275 Fahrenheit.
8. Serve and enjoy it.

NUTRITION: Calories: 286 cal Fat: 14 g Protein: 7 g Carbs: 36 g

4.4. Fresh Fruit Pizza

Ready in: 20 minutes

Servings: 10

Difficulty: Easy

INGREDIENTS

Dough

- 2 tsp vanilla extract
- 1 2/3 cups all-purpose flour
- ¼ tsp baking soda
- ½ tsp baking powder
- ¼ tsp salt
- 12 tbsp butter
- ¾ cup sugar
- One egg

Cream cheese topping

- 6 tbsp sugar
- 8 oz cream cheese
- ½ tsp vanilla extract

Fruit layer

- ¼ cup apricot
- 5 cups chopped fruits, fresh
- 1 tbsp water

DIRECTIONS

1. Combine baking powder, salt, flour, and baking soda in a bowl and whisk well.
2. Blend butter with sugar using an electric mixer to get a smooth mixture.
3. Now add egg and vanilla extract in butter mixture and blend again.
4. Stir in flour and blend again.
5. Transfer the batter into a pizza pan lined with parchment paper and evenly spread it.
6. Bake for 15 minutes in a preheated oven at 350 Fahrenheit.
7. After 15 minutes, take it out of the oven and let it cool down.
8. Blend cream cheese, sugar, and vanilla extract in a blender to form cream cheese topping for the curst.
9. Spread the cream cheese mixture evenly over the baked crust.
10. Now, garnish pizza with fruits.
11. Serve and enjoy it.

NUTRITION: Calories: 450 cal Fat: 22 g Protein: 5 g Carbs: 59 g

4.5. Tomato Omelets

Ready in: 30 minutes

Servings: 4

Difficulty: Medium

INGREDIENTS

- One pinch of garam masala
- 1 cup gram flour
- One chopped onion
- Two chopped tomatoes
- One pinch of hing
- ½ inch chopped ginger
- ¼ cup chopped cilantro
- One chopped green chili
- ¼ tsp red chili powder
- ¼ tsp turmeric powder
- Salt as needed
- ½ cup water
- Oil as required

DIRECTIONS

1. Combine basin, onions, coriander, ginger, chili, and tomatoes in a bowl.
2. Mix in all the spices and add water.
3. Mix everything well to get a smooth batter. The batter should have a medium consistency.
4. Heat oil in a pan over medium flame.

5. Pour the batter into the pan using a spoon and spread it over the pan's whole surface. You can rotate the pan for spreading the batter.
6. After 2 minutes, drizzle oil over the top of the batter and flip it to cook the other side of the omelet.
7. Transfer the omelet to the serving plate.
8. Serve and enjoy it.

NUTRITION: Calories: 217 cal Fat: 15 g Protein: 6 g Carbs: 19 g

4.6. Chilaquiles with Gochujang

Ready in: 30 minutes

Servings: 4

Difficulty: Medium

INGREDIENTS

- 1 tbsp olive oil
- One dried Ancho Chile
- 5 cups tortilla chips
- 1 cup tomatoes, crushed
- 2 cups water
- Two garlic cloves
- 1 ½ tbsp gochujang
- 1 tsp salt
- Three eggs

Toppings

- avocado
- Cilantro
- Onions
- Jalapeno peppers

DIRECTIONS

1. Add water to the pan and let it boil over a high flame.
2. Mix in ancho chile in boiling water and let it rest there for 15 minutes so that it can get plump up.
3. Extract chile using tongs. Save water for further use.

4. Add soaked chile, hot water, tomatoes, salt, garlic, and gochujang in a blender and blend to get a smooth mixture.
5. Transfer the mixture to saucepan and heat for five minutes over medium flame.
6. Remove the pan from the flame and add tortilla pieces. Mix well.
7. Heat oil in a pan and fry eggs one by one and transfer them to the plate.
8. Transfer the tortillas dipped in sauce in the serving dish and garnished cilantro, onions, fried egg, and avocado.
9. Serve and enjoy it.

NUTRITION: Calories: 407 cal Fat: 21 g Protein: 12.5 g Carbs: 44 g

4.7. French Toast

Ready in: 30 minutes

Servings: 4

Difficulty: Medium

INGREDIENTS

- ½ cup maple syrup
- 1 tsp cinnamon
- 2 tbsp sugar
- Eight bread slices
- ¼ tsp nutmeg
- 4 tbsp butter
- ¼ cup milk
- Four eggs
- ½ tsp vanilla extract

DIRECTIONS

1. Mix sugar, cinnamon, and nutmeg in a bowl and keep the bowl aside for a while.
2. Now whisk egg, vanilla, and milk in a cinnamon mixture.
3. Dip each slice of bread in an egg and cinnamon mixture.
4. Fry egg dipped bread slices in melted butter in a skillet over medium flame.
5. Fry the sliced from both sides until turned golden.
6. Serve and enjoy it.

NUTRITION: Calories: 95 cal Fat: 3 g Protein: 4 g Carbs: 13 g

4.8. Blueberry Muffins

Ready in: 30 minutes

Servings: 4

Difficulty: Medium

INGREDIENTS

- 7 oz fresh blueberries
- 1 ½ cups all-purpose flour
- ¼ tsp salt
- ¾ cup sugar
- 2 tsp baking powder
- ½ cup milk
- 1/3 cup canola oil
- 1 ½ tsp vanilla extract

DIRECTIONS

1. Combine salt, sugar, flour, and baking powder in a mixing bowl and whisk well.
2. Whisk oil, egg, milk, and vanilla in another container and mix well to combine everything evenly.
3. Now, mix the liquid mixture with the dry mixture.
4. Transfer the batter in muffin cups lined with parchment paper.
5. Garnish the top with sugar.
6. Bake in a preheated oven at 400 Fahrenheit for 20 minutes.
7. Serve and enjoy it.

NUTRITION: Calories: 217 cal Fat: 8 g Protein: 3 g Carbs: 33 g

Chapter 5: Smoothies and Drinks Recipes

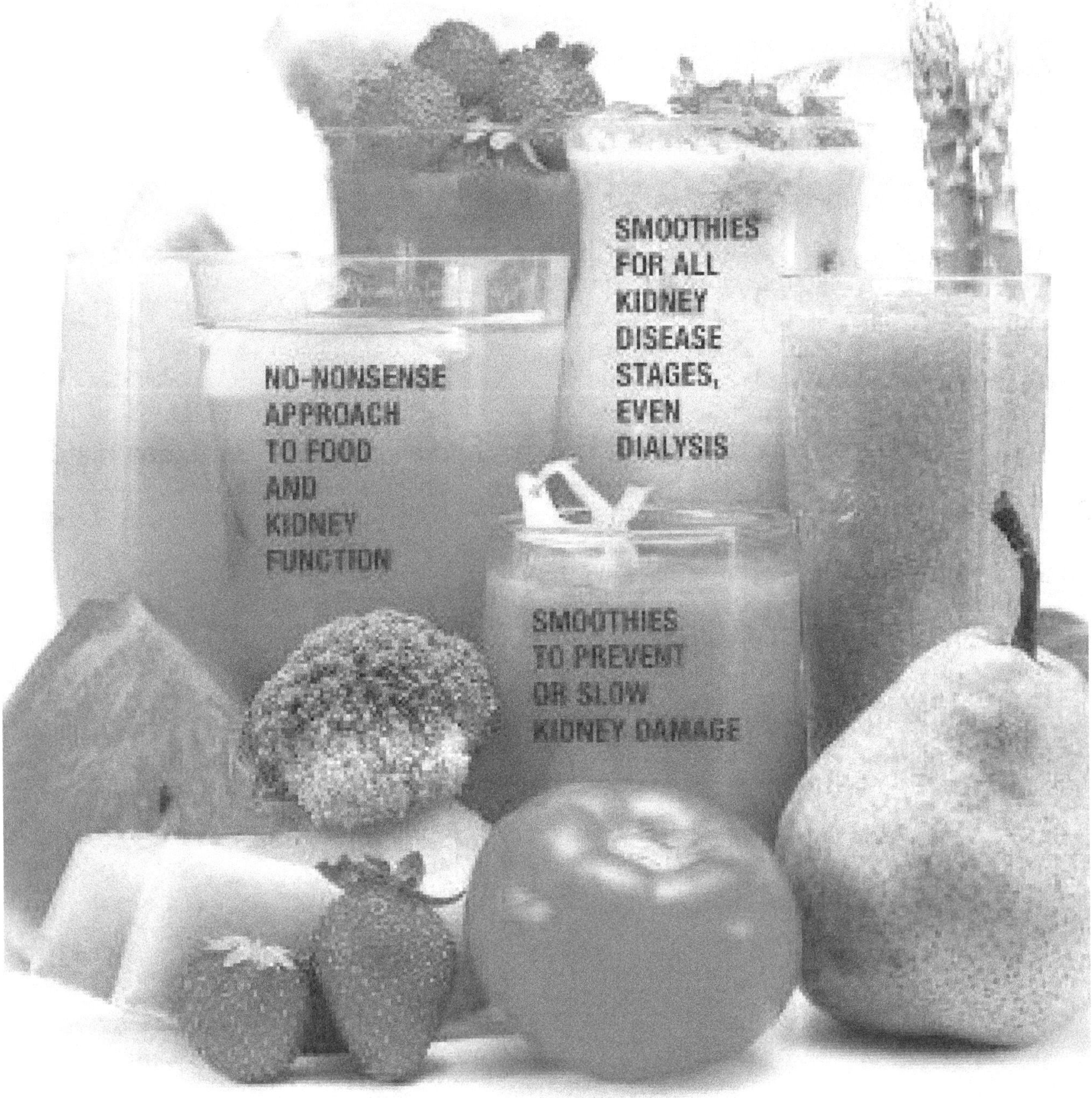

5.1. Blue Hawaii Smoothie

Ready in: 3 minutes

Servings: 3

Difficulty: Easy

INGREDIENTS

- One banana
- Two ¼ cup blueberries, frozen
- 2 cups pineapple juice
- Eight ice cubes

DIRECTIONS

1. Add all the ingredients to a food processor and blend to get a smooth mixture.
2. Transfer the mixture to serving glass.
3. Serve and enjoy it.

NUTRITION: Calories: 220 cal Fat: 3 g Protein: 5 g Carbs: 43 g

5.2. Lemon and ginger green juice

Ready in: 20 minutes

Servings: 4

Difficulty: Easy

INGREDIENTS

- Two lemons, peeled
- One sliced cucumber
- ½ inch ginger, peeled
- One celery head stalks separated
- One diced green apple

DIRECTIONS

1. Wash all the ingredients and chop them.
2. Add ginger, cucumber, lemons, celery, and apple in a juicer and squeeze to extract their juice.
3. Transfer the juice to the serving glasses.
4. Serve and enjoy it.
5. If not using immediately, pour it into an airtight container and place it in the fridge.
6. Use it within 24 hours of preparation to avoid its spoiled taste.

NUTRITION: Calories: 63 cal Fat: 0.3 g Protein: 1 g Carbs: 17.6 g

5.3. Pineapple Juice

Ready in: 10 minutes

Servings: 2

Difficulty: Easy

INGREDIENTS

- ¼ tsp black salt
- 3 cups pineapple, fresh
- 2 tbsp sugar
- 1 cup water
- Ice cubes as required

DIRECTIONS

1. Remove the skin peeling off the pineapple and dice it.
2. Place diced pieces of pineapple in a food processor.
3. Add sugar and water to a food processor and blend to obtain the smooth texture juice of pineapple.
4. Transfer the juice to the glass after straining it.
5. At this point, you can adjust the consistency of the juice by adding water to it.
6. Add ice cubes in serving glasses.
7. Transfer the juice to ice cubed glasses.
8. Drizzle powdered black pepper over each glass.
9. Put pineapple wedge over the side of the glass and sprinkle mint at the top.
10. Serve and enjoy it.

NUTRITION: Calories: 795 kcal Fat: 1 g Protein: 5 g Carbs: 193 g

5.4. Grapefruit Sorbet

Ready in: 40 minutes

Servings: 6

Difficulty: Medium

INGREDIENTS

- 1 ½ cup grapefruit juice
- One ¼ cups water
- 1 tbsp zest of grapefruit
- 1 cup sugar

DIRECTIONS

1. Add water to a pot and let it boil over a high flame.
2. Add sugar and mix well.
3. Cook until all the sugar is fully dissolved in the water. The sugary syrup is ready.
4. Turn off the flame and mix in grapefruit zest and keep it aside to cool it down.
5. When it is fully cooled down, pour in grapefruit juice and mix well.
6. Cover the pot with a lid and place it in the fridge for four hours to chill it.
7. After four hours, transfer the chilled mixture to the ice cream maker.
8. Churn the ice maker to get a creamy smooth-textured mixture.
9. Serve and enjoy it.
10. You can also store it in the fridge for later use.

NUTRITION: Calories: 116.1 cal Fat: 0.1 g Protein: 0.3 g Carbs: 30.2 g

5.5. Watermelon Granita

Ready in: 30 minutes

Servings: 8

Difficulty: Medium

INGREDIENTS

- 3 tbsp lime juice
- 2 tbsp coconut sugar
- 2 lb sliced watermelon

DIRECTIONS

1. Add coconut sugar, diced watermelon, and lime juice to the food processor.
2. Blend to get a smooth mixture.
3. Transfer the mixture to the pan and place the pan for two hours in the freezer.
4. After two hours of freezing, scrape the freezing mixture using a spatula and break the ice crystals. The mixture should have a flaky slushy look.
5. You can also add the mixture to the blender and blend to get creamy smooth-textured granite.
6. Transfer the granite to the serving dish.
7. Serve and enjoy it.
8. You want to store it, cover the granite with a placed sheet, cover the pot with a lid and place it in the freezer.
9. You can store it for seven days.

NUTRITION: Calories: 50 cal Fat: 0 g Protein: 0 g Carbs: 14 g

5.6. Banana Breeze Pie

Ready in: 30 minutes

Servings: 5

Difficulty: Medium

INGREDIENTS

Cracker crust

- ½ cup butter
- ¼ cup sugar
- 1 ½ cups graham crackers crumbs

Filling for Pie

- ¼ cup sugar, powdered
- Four bananas
- 14 oz condensed milk
- 8 oz cream cheese
- 1/3 cup lemon juice
- Whipping cream
- ½ tbsp vanilla extract
- 1 cup heavy cream

DIRECTIONS

Graham Cracker Crust

1. Add whole graham crackers in a blender and blend to get fine powdered cracker crumbs.
2. Transfer the cracker crumbs to a bowl.

3. Mix in melted butter and sugar. Mix well.
4. Shift the cracker crumbs mixture in the pan. Press using your hands to make it firm, layer in the pan, and distribute it evenly.
5. Cover the pan with a plastic sheet and put it in the freezer until further use.

Pie Filling

1. Whisk cream cheese using an electric mixer to get a creamy smooth-textured mixture.
2. Stir in condensed milk, vanilla extract, and lemon juice and whisk well. The pie filling is ready to be used.
3. Peel the bananas and slice them.
4. Make a layer of banana slices over the crust. Make sure to cover the crust of the pie with banana slices completely.
5. Transfer the pie filling to the curst.
6. Spread the filling evenly over the crust and place the pan in the freezer for five hours while covering the top with a plastic sheet.

Whipping cream

1. Combine sugar and heavy cream in a cold mixing bowl and beat using an electric beater for 10 minutes to get stiff peaks.
2. Pour the whipped cream into a bag with a nozzle at the end.
3. Now using the nozzle decorate the pie top accordingly.
4. Garnish the top with banana slices. You can swirl whipped cream too over the banana slices.
5. Serve and enjoy it.

NUTRITION: Calories: 420.4 cal Fat: 22 g Protein: 7.1 g Carbs: 52 g

5.7. Kidney nourishing smoothie

Ready in: 5 minutes

Servings: 2

Difficulty: Easy

INGREDIENTS

- 1 cup ice
- 1.2 sliced cucumber
- 1 cup coconut water
- 1 cup blueberries, fresh
- 2 tbsp chia seeds
- 2 tbsp of lime juice
- Stevia as required
- One pinch of cinnamon

DIRECTIONS

1. Combine cucumber, blueberries, cinnamon, water, ice, chia seeds, stevia, and lime juice in a food processor.
2. Blend to speed and then run the food processor at high speed.
3. Keep it blending for more than one minute.
4. When you see that everything is blended perfectly and have achieved the required consistency, turn off the machine.
5. Transfer the smoothie into serving glasses.
6. Garnish with favorite toppings.
7. Serve and enjoy it.

NUTRITION: Calories: 70 cal Fat: 0.5 g Protein: 0.3 g Carbs: 16.5 g

5.8. Mixed berry protein smoothie

Ready in: 5 minutes

Servings: 1

Difficulty: Easy

INGREDIENTS

- 1 tsp vanilla extract
- ¼ cup water
- ¼ cup yogurt
- ½ cup mixed berries
- ¼ cup oats
- 1 tsp honey
- 1 tbsp vanilla protein powder

DIRECTIONS

1. Combine protein powder, berries, vanilla extract, sliced oats, water, honey, and plain greek yogurt in the food processor,
2. Blend to obtain a creamy-textured smooth mixture.
3. Transfer the creamy mixture into the serving dish.
4. Garnish it.
5. Serve and enjoy it.

NUTRITION: Calories: 398 cal Fat: 6 g Protein: 28 g Carbs: 59 g

Chapter 6: Snacks and Sides Recipes

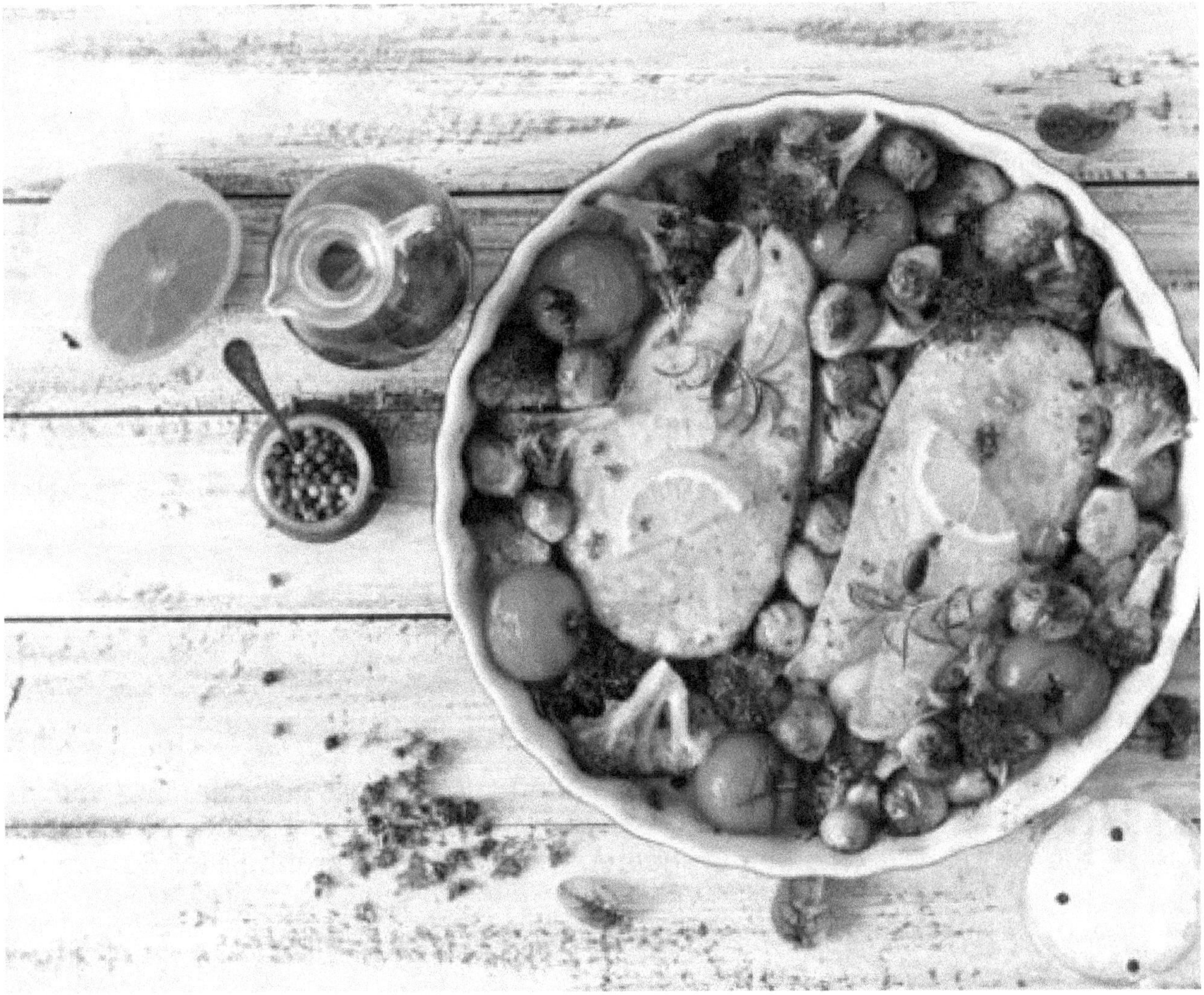

6.1. Baba Ganoush

Ready in: 55 minutes

Servings: 6

Difficulty: Medium

INGREDIENTS

- ¼ tsp paprika, smoked
- 2 lb eggplants
- 2 tbsp lemon juice
- ¾ tsp salt
- Two minced garlic cloves
- ¼ cup tahini
- 2 tbsp chopped parsley, fresh
- 1/3 cup olive oil
- ¼ tsp cumin

DIRECTIONS

1. Slice the eggplants into two halves and rub olive oil on each side.
2. Place the halves of the eggplant in a baking tray lined with parchment paper.
3. Bake the eggplant halves in a preheated oven at 450 Fahrenheit for 35 minutes.
4. Remove the eggplant from the oven and let them cool down.
5. Take out the flesh from the eggplant using a spoon and place the flesh in a bowl. Keep the bowl aside for a while to allow the eggplant to release the maximum moisture.
6. Abandon the dripping of the eggplant.
7. Stir in lemon juice, tahini, olive oil, and garlic in eggplant and vigorously stir to blend everything well.

8. Mix in salt, parsley, and cumin, and toss well.
9. Shift baba ganoush to the serving container.
10. Drizzle oil, paprika, and parsley over baba ganoush.
11. Serve and enjoy it.

NUTRITION: Calories: 248 cal Fat: 23 g Protein: 3.3 g Carbs: 12 g

6.2. Hot Crab Dip

Ready in: 25 minutes

Servings: 4

Difficulty: Easy

INGREDIENTS

- Black pepper to taste
- 8 oz cream cheese
- ¼ tsp paprika, smoked
- ½ cup mayonnaise
- ½ cup parmesan cheese, grated
- 12 oz white crab meat
- Two chopped onions, green
- Salt to taste

DIRECTIONS

1. Whisk paprika, cream cheese, and mayo in a bowl to get a smooth mixture.
2. Mix in cheese, crab, salt, green onion, and pepper, and toss well.
3. Transfer the mixture to a baking tray.
4. Bake in a preheated oven at 350 Fahrenheit for 10 minutes.
5. After 10 minutes, sprinkle parmesan cheese and bake again to melt the cheese.
6. Serve and enjoy it.

NUTRITION: Calories: 506 cal Fat: 44 g Protein: 23 g Carbs: 3 g

6.3. Aubergine and Chickpea Bites

Ready in: 70 minutes

Servings: 20

Difficulty: Medium

INGREDIENTS

- 3 tbsp polenta
- Three aubergines, sliced
- 2 tsp coriander
- Two peeled garlic cloves
- 2 tsp cumin seeds
- 2 tbsp gram flour
- 3 ½ cup chickpeas
- 1 tbsp lemon zest
- One wedge cut lemon slices
- 1 tbsp lemon juice

Dipping sauce

- 1 ½ cup coconut yogurt
- 1 tbsp harissa

DIRECTIONS

1. Spread olive oil over the slices of Aubergine.
2. Put the aubergine slices in a baking tray.
3. Sprinkle garlic, salt, cumin, pepper, and coriander over Aubergine.
4. Bake in a preheated oven at 200 Fahrenheit for 40 minutes.
5. After 40 minutes, remove Aubergine and let it cool down.

6. Take out the flesh of Aubergine and throw away the skin.
7. Mesh the flesh of Aubergine, garlic, and spices using a spoon.
8. Stir in gram flour, juice, chickpeas, and lemon zest and toss well.
9. Make ball shapes out of the batter and place them in a baking dish covered with butter paper.
10. Place the dish in the fridge for 25 minutes.
11. Meanwhile, whisk yogurt and harissa in a bowl and set aside until further use.
12. Add polenta to a flat dish.
13. Coat balls in polenta and spray them with oil
14. Bake in a preheated oven at 200 Fahrenheit for 20 minutes.
15. Serve and enjoy it with harissa sauce.

NUTRITION: Calories: 66 kcal Fat: 3 g Protein: 2 g Carbs: 6 g

6.4. Date and Walnut Porridge

Ready in: 10 minutes

Servings: 1

Difficulty: Easy

INGREDIENTS

- ½ cup strawberries
- 2 ½ cup milk
- 1/3 cup buckwheat flakes
- Four chopped walnuts
- One chopped date
- 1 tsp walnut butter

DIRECTIONS

1. Add dates and milk to a pot and let them heat for three minutes.
2. Stir in buckwheat flakes and mix well.
3. Let it cook until the consistency to the desired level is achieved.
4. Add walnut butter and toss well.
5. Sprinkle walnuts and strawberries.
6. Serve and enjoy it.

NUTRITION: Calories: 229 kcal Fat: 23 g Protein: 16 g Carbs: 66 g

6.5. Tuna Egg Salad with Rice, Capers, and Cucumbers

Ready in: 30 minutes

Servings: 3

Difficulty: Easy

INGREDIENTS

- Black pepper to taste
- One chopped yellow onion
- 1 cup tuna
- 3 tbsp mayonnaise
- Two chopped boiled eggs
- 1 cup white rice, cooked
- Two diced cucumbers
- 2 tbsp capers
- Salt to taste

DIRECTIONS

1. Add black pepper, onion, tuna, capers, salt, cooked rice, mayonnaise, boiled eggs, and cucumber in a large mixing bowl and toss well.
2. Serve and enjoy it.
3. You can use it as a spread over bread or capers.

NUTRITION: Calories: 335 cal Fat: 15 g Protein: 23 g Carbs: 23 g

6.6. Caramelized banana and ginger snap parfaits

Ready in: 10 minutes

Servings: 2

Difficulty: Easy

INGREDIENTS

- Cassonade syrup to taste
- Two sliced bananas
- 16 oz greek yogurt
- 3 tbsp brown sugar
- Gingersnap cookies

DIRECTIONS

1. Place sugar on a plate and roll peeled bananas in the sugar to coat it properly.
2. Heat oil in a pan over medium flame.
3. Place coated bananas in the pan and cook for five minutes.
4. After five minutes, change the bananas' direction by carefully flipping them—Cook for three minutes.
5. Transfer the cooked sugar-coated bananas to the plate and keep them aside.
6. Make a layer of yogurt in the jar, followed by cooked bananas, crumbled cookies, and cassonade syrup.
7. Repeat the process.
8. Serve and enjoy it.
9. You can also keep it in the refrigerator and eat it later on.

NUTRITION: Calories: 370 cal Fat: 5 g Protein: 8.2 g Carbs: 70.5 g

6.7. Marshmallow Popcorn Balls

Ready in: 30 minutes

Servings: 8

Difficulty: Medium

INGREDIENTS

- 5 cups marshmallows
- 1 tbsp vegetable oil
- 6 tbsp butter
- ½ cup popcorn, unpopped

DIRECTIONS

1. Heat oil in a skillet over a high flame.
2. Add popping corn and constantly stir them.
3. When popcorns are done, transfer them to the plate and keep them aside until further use.
4. Now, add butter to a pan and melt it over low flame.
5. Add marshmallows and constantly stir them until fully melted.
6. Transfer the melted marshmallows over the cooked popcorns and toss well to coat popcorns with marshmallow syrup.
7. Place the mixture aside to cool them.
8. Make balls of the required size and place them in a serving bowl.
9. Serve and enjoy it.

NUTRITION: Calories: 273 cal Fat: 11 g Protein: 2.2 g Carbs: 34.7 g

6.8. **Hummus**

Ready in: 10 minutes

Servings: 8

Difficulty: Easy

INGREDIENTS

- Two smashed garlic cloves
- 1/3 cup tahini
- 2 tbsp olive oil
- 4 tbsp cold water
- ½ tsp cumin
- 3 tbsp lemon juice
- Olive oil for topping
- 15 oz chickpeas
- Parsley, chopped for topping
- ¾ tsp salt

DIRECTIONS

1. Combine olive oil, salt, lemon juice, tahini, garlic, cold water, and cumin in a blender and blend to get a smooth puree.
2. Now put chickpeas in the same blender and blend with tahini mixture. Keep on scraping down the mixture from the sides of the blender walls so that everything is blended properly and you get a smooth texture puree of chickpeas. If the mixture has a thick consistency, you can add water or olive oil according to your taste to reduce the consistency.
3. At this point, you can adjust the taste accordingly by adding cumin, salt, or lemon juice.

4. Transfer the puree to a serving dish.
5. Make a well at the center of the hummus and pour olive oil.
6. Sprinkle red chilies or your favorite toppings.
7. Serve and enjoy it.
8. You can store it for three days by putting it in an airtight container and place it in the fridge.

NUTRITION: Calories: 176 cal Fat: 8.7 g Protein: 7.2 g Carbs: 19.4 g

Chapter 7: Soup Recipes

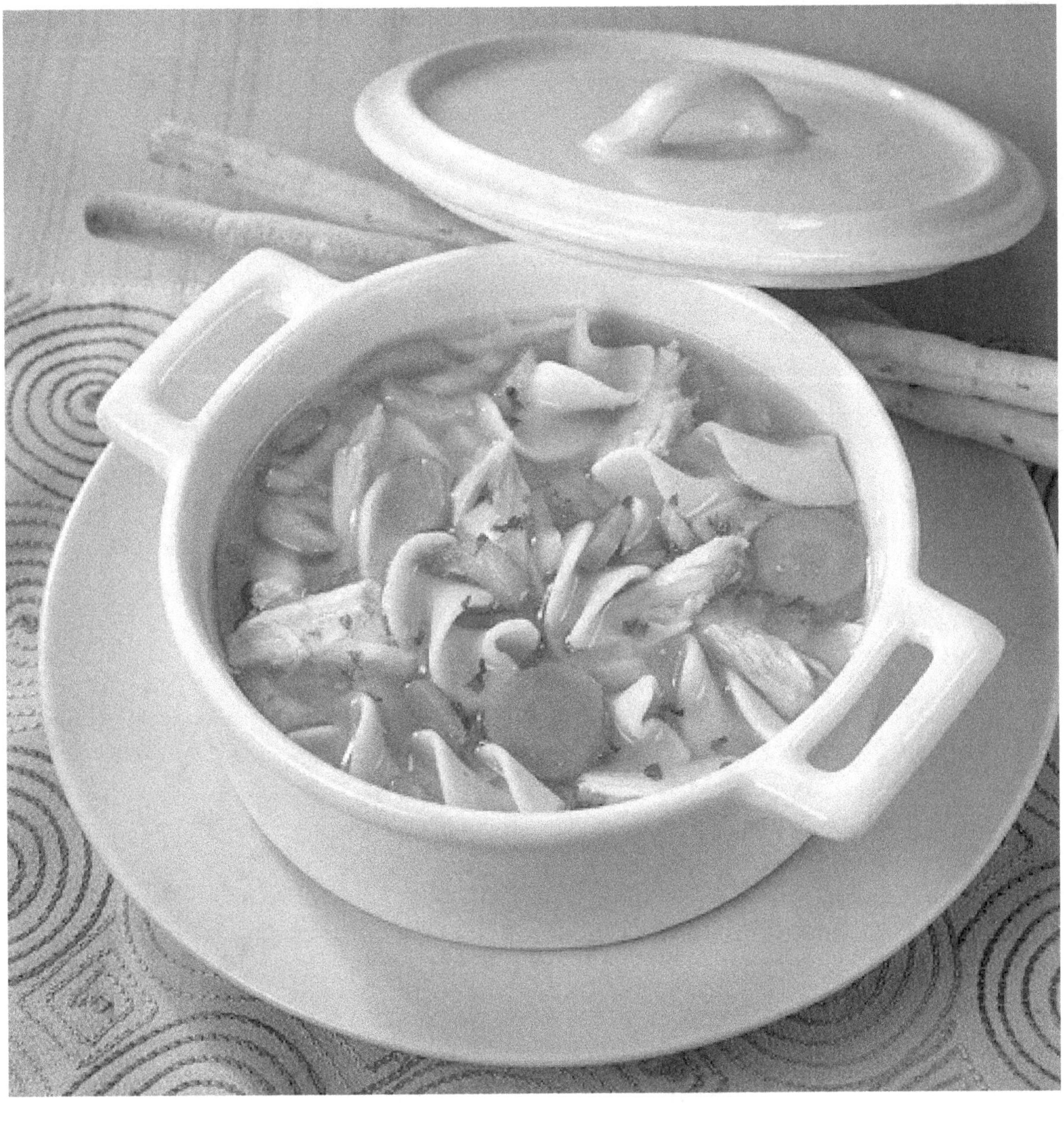

7.1. French Onion Soup

Ready in: 60 minutes

Servings: 5

Difficulty: Medium

INGREDIENTS

- Salt to taste
- 4 lb sliced yellow onions
- Four minced garlic cloves
- 3 tbsp butter
- 3 tbsp flour
- Baguette
- 6 cups beef stock
- ½ cup white wine, dry
- One bay leaf
- Grated cheese as required
- 1 tsp Worcestershire sauce
- 1 tsp thyme, dried
- Black pepper to taste

DIRECTIONS

1. Sauté onions in heated butter in a skillet over medium flame.
2. Fry onions until caramelized for about 30 minutes with occasional stirring.
3. Stir in garlic and cook for three minutes.
4. Now add flour and mix.

5. Cook for one more minute with constant stirring.
6. Pour in the wine and stir and cook.
7. Pour in bay leaf, thyme, Worcestershire, and stock and mix well.
8. Let it simmer and cover the pan, reduce the flame to low, and cook for 10 minutes.
9. After 10 minutes, add pepper and salt according to the taste.
10. Place the sliced baguette in the baking tray in a single layer.
11. Bake in a preheated oven at 400 Fahrenheit for 8 minutes.
12. Transfer the crisp baguette pieces to the plate and keep them aside.
13. Pour the soup into a serving oven-safe bowl.
14. Add baguette pieces and cheese.
15. Place the bowl in the oven at broil mode and let it broil for five minutes.
16. Serve and enjoy it.

NUTRITION: Calories: 618 cal Fat: 27 g Protein: 26 g Carbs: 59 g

7.2. Turkey Bulgur Soup

Ready in: 70 minutes

Servings: 6

Difficulty: Medium

INGREDIENTS

- Black pepper to taste
- 1 tsp olive oil
- ½ chopped sweet onion
- ½ lb turkey, cooked
- 1 tsp chopped sage, fresh
- 4 cups water
- 1 tsp chopped garlic
- 1/3 tsp red pepper flakes
- 1 cup chicken stock
- One sliced carrot
- 2 tbsp chopped parsley, fresh
- One chopped celery stalk
- ½ cup shredded cabbage
- Two bay leaves, dried
- ½ cup bulgur
- 1 tsp chopped thyme, fresh

DIRECTIONS

1. Heat olive oil over medium flame in a pan.
2. Add turkey and cook for five minutes.

3. Stir in garlic and onion and sauté for four minutes.
4. Pour in cabbage, water, celery, bay leaves, stock, carrot, and bulgur and mix well.
5. Let it boil and decrease the flame.
6. Let the soup boil for 35 minutes.
7. Take away the bay leaves and mix in sage, pepper flakes, black pepper, parsley, and thyme.
8. Serve and enjoy it.

NUTRITION: Calories: 124 kcal Fat: 5 g Protein: 11 g Carbs: 8 g

7.3. Italian Sausage Soup

Ready in: 50 minutes

Servings: 10

Difficulty: Medium

INGREDIENTS

- ½ tsp black pepper
- 1 lb ground Italian sausage
- ½ chopped red pepper
- ½ cup chopped onion
- 2 tsp mashed garlic
- 2 tbsp flour
- 2 tbsp butter
- 6 cups chicken broth
- 2 cups half-n-half cream
- 12 oz egg noodles
- 3 cups spinach
- ½ cup parmesan cheese grated

DIRECTIONS

1. Cook sausage in a pot over medium flame.
2. Transfer the sausage to a paper towel and pat to remove extra fat and place them on a plate and keep it aside.
3. Melt butter in the same pan over medium flame.
4. Sauté red pepper, onions, and garlic for five minutes.
5. Stir in flour and mix to coat—Cook for a minute with constant stirring.

6. Pour in chicken stock and let it boil.

7. Add egg noodles and let it cook with occasional stirring for 21 minutes.

8. Mix in cream, sausage, and spinach, and cook for 10 minutes.

9. Sprinkle pepper and grated cheese. Toss well.

10. Serve and enjoy it.

NUTRITION: Calories: 324 cal Fat: 22 g Protein: 15 g Carbs: 17 g

7.4. Vietnamese Chicken Pho Soup

Ready in: 100 minutes

Servings: 5

Difficulty: Medium

INGREDIENTS

Charred aromatics

- Two onions
- 1 tbsp oil
- 3 tbsp sliced ginger

Pho soup broth

- ¾ tsp salt
- 8 cups water
- ½ cup cilantro
- 3 lb chicken thigh
- 6 tsp white sugar
- 5-star anise pods
- Four garlic cloves
- One cinnamon stick
- 2 tsp fennel seeds
- 8 tsp fish sauce
- 2 tsp coriander seeds

Noodle bowl

- Two sliced green onions
- 13 oz rice noodles

Toppings

- Two wedges cut lines
- 1/3 cup coriander
- 3 cups bean sprouts

Hoisin sauce

- Red chilies
- Sriracha

DIRECTIONS

1. Add oil to a large pot and heat it over a high flame.
2. Add onion and ginger and leave them for five minutes by turning them halfway.
3. Mix in coriander seeds, anise pods, garlic, fennel seeds, cinnamon sticks, water, cilantro, sugar, fish sauce, and chicken thigh.
4. Let it simmer and cover the pot for 70 minutes.
5. Strain the soup in another clean pot and separate the chicken pieces.
6. Now sprinkle salt and mix well. Keep it aside until further use.
7. Now cook noodles as per the instructions written over the packet.
8. Transfer the cooked noodles to the bowl and add chicken and broth.
9. Spread green onions at the top.
10. You can add your favorite toppings over the soup and add lime juice to enhance the taste.
11. Serve and enjoy it.

NUTRITION: Calories: 501 cal Fat: 8 g Protein: 20 g Carbs: 87 g

7.5. Golden beet soup

Ready in: 90 minutes

Servings: 8

Difficulty: Medium

INGREDIENTS

- 3 tbsp lemon juice
- 6 tbsp pareve margarine
- 1 tbsp lemon peel
- 4 ½ cups diced onions
- 9 cups sliced golden beets
- 4 tsp smashed ginger
- 6 cups chicken broth

DIRECTIONS

1. Heat margarine over medium flame in the pot.
2. Sauté onions, lemon peels, beets, and ginger in heated margarine for 15 minutes with occasional stirring.
3. Pour in the stock and let it boil.
4. Cover the pot and decrease the flame to low, and cook it for 60 minutes.
5. After one hour, remove the pot from the flame and let it cool down completely.
6. Pour the soup into a food processor and blend to get a smooth solution.
7. Now transfer the blend soup solution to the pot and cook it.
8. Add lemon juice, pepper, and salt and stir.
9. You can adjust the consistency of the soup at this point by adding more stock solution.
10. Steam the beet greens to wilt them.

11. Add wilt beet greens in a blender with one cup of soup.

12. Blend them to obtain a smooth solution.

13. Serve soup with beet green puree and enjoy it.

NUTRITION: Calories: 157 cal Fat: 5.2 g Protein: 3.5 g Carbs: 28 g

7.6. Sopa da lima

Ready in: 45 minutes

Servings: 8

Difficulty: Medium

INGREDIENTS

- 1 ½ lb chicken breast, boneless
- Eight corn tortillas
- Salt to taste
- One chopped tomato
- ½ cup vegetable oil
- One chopped onion
- One sliced carrot
- One chopped avocado
- One sliced celery rib
- One chopped jalapeno
- 1/3 cup lime juice
- One bay leaf
- Four minced garlic cloves
- ¼ tsp oregano, dried
- 8 cups chicken stock
- Two chopped onions
- 2 tbsp chopped cilantro, fresh

DIRECTIONS

1. Heat oil in a skillet over medium heat.
2. Slice the tortillas and fry them in heated oil for a minute to have crisp and golden tortillas.
3. Sprinkle salt and place them on a plate. Keep the plate aside until further use.
4. Heat oil again in a skillet over medium flame.
5. Sauté carrot, onion, jalapeno pepper, and celery for five minutes with occasional stirring.
6. Stir in oregano, bay leaf, and garlic, and cook for a minute.
7. Mix in salt and tomato and cook for five minutes.
8. Pour in chicken pieces and chicken broth and let it boil.
9. Decrease the flame to low and let it simmer for 15 minutes.
10. After 15 minutes of simmering, take out the chicken pieces and keep the soup on the flame to simmer for some more time.
11. Shred the boiled chicken into small pieces and add the shredded chicken pieces back to the soup pot.
12. Mix in lime juice and sliced green onions and cook for seven more minutes.
13. Adjust the taste of the soup accordingly by adding pepper and salt.
14. Pour the soup into serving bowls and top it with tortillas.
15. Sprinkle cilantro and avocado pieces.
16. Serve and enjoy it.

NUTRITION: Calories: 378 cal Fat: 22 g Protein: 26 g Carbs: 21 g

7.7. Chicken soup base

Ready in: 55 minutes

Servings: 8

Difficulty: Medium

INGREDIENTS

- 1 tsp thyme leaves, dried
- 8 cups chicken broth
- 2 lb chicken
- Two sliced celery stalk
- 4 cups water
- 3 tbsp vegetable oil
- Two diced carrots
- Two diced onions

DIRECTIONS

1. Add water and stock in a pot over medium flame and bring it to simmer.
2. Remove the bones and skin from the chicken pieces and add them to the pot.
3. Cover the pot and decrease the flame.
4. Let it simmer for 25 minutes.
5. Strain the soup and keep it aside.
6. Heat oil in the same pot over medium flame.
7. Sauté carrot, onions, and celery for 10 minutes.
8. Stir in broth, chicken, and thyme and let it simmer for 10 minutes.
9. Transfer the soup to the serving bowl.
10. Serve and enjoy it.

NUTRITION: Calories: 338 cal Fat: 21.3 g Protein: 30 g Carbs: 5.8 g

7.8. Mushroom Broth Soup

Ready in: 55 minutes

Servings: 5

Difficulty: Medium

INGREDIENTS

- 1 tbsp sliced green onions
- One ¾ cups beef broth
- 1/8 tsp black pepper
- ¼ cup sliced celery
- One ¾ cups chicken broth
- 1/8 tsp crushed rosemary leaves, dried
- ¼ cup sliced carrot
- 2 cups sliced mushrooms
- One chopped onion
- ¼ cup peas

DIRECTIONS

1. Add black pepper, carrot, beef, chicken stock, onion, rosemary, peas, mushrooms, and celery over medium flames in a large pot.
2. Cover the pot and decrease the flame to low, and let it cook for 18 minutes.
3. Stir in chopped green onions and cook for seven minutes.
4. Transfer the soup to the serving bowl.
5. Serve and enjoy it.

NUTRITION: Calories: 81 cal Fat: 3.8 g Protein: 4.6 g Carbs: 9.6 g

Chapter 8: Salad Recipes

8.1. Honey Roasted walnuts

Ready in: 20 minutes

Servings: 1

Difficulty: Easy

INGREDIENTS

- 1 tsp salt
- 1 cup walnuts
- ¼ cup sugar
- 2 tbsp honey
- ½ tsp chili powder

DIRECTIONS

1. Combine sugar, walnuts, salt, honey, and chili powder in a bowl and toss well.
2. Transfer the walnut mixture into the baking tray lined with parchment paper and spread it.
3. Bake in a preheated oven at 350 Fahrenheit for 20 minutes with the occasional turning of the walnuts.
4. Serve and enjoy it.

NUTRITION: Calories: 475 kcal Fat: 76 g Protein: 18 g Carbs: 205 g

8.2. Basil Walnut Pesto

Ready in: 10 minutes

Servings: 10

Difficulty: Easy

INGREDIENTS

- Black pepper as required
- 2 cups basil leaves, fresh
- One mashed garlic clove
- ¼ cup walnuts
- 1 tsp lemon juice
- Salt to taste
- 1/3 cup olive oil

DIRECTIONS

1. Combine basil, lemon juice. Olive oil, walnuts, and garlic in a food processor.
2. Blend to obtain a smooth mixture.
3. Sprinkle black pepper and salt to adjust the taste. Toss well. The pesto is ready.
4. If you want to store it for longer, pour the pesto into a jar and fill it with olive oil.
5. You can also freeze it and can use it in stew or soup.

NUTRITION: Calories: 93 cal Fat: 10 g Protein: 0 g Carbs: 1 g

8.3. Artichoke arugula salad with parmesan

Ready in: 20 minutes

Servings: 4

Difficulty: Easy

INGREDIENTS

- 1/3 cup grated parmesan
- 8 cups arugula
- 9 oz artichoke hearts, frozen and thawed
- Salt to taste
- 2 tbsp olive oil
- 2 tbsp wine vinegar
- 1 tsp Dijon mustard
- Black pepper as required
- 1 lb sliced bulb fennel

DIRECTIONS

1. Heat oil in a skillet over medium flame.
2. Add salt, artichokes, and black pepper and stir well.
3. Place the skillet in preheated broiler and let it broil for seven minutes.
4. Transfer the cooked artichokes to a bowl and keep them aside.
5. Add arugula and fennel in artichoke and toss well.
6. Combine salt, vinegar, olive oil, water, black pepper, and mustard in a container and toss well.
7. Mix vinegar mixture with artichoke mixture.
8. Sprinkle cheese and serve.

9. Enjoy it.

NUTRITION: Calories: 147 cal Fat: 10 g Protein: 6 g Carbs: 11 g

8.4. Italian Tomato Cucumber Salad

Ready in: 10 minutes

Servings: 4

Difficulty: Easy

INGREDIENTS

- ¼ cup Italian salad dressing
- Two sliced cucumbers
- One chopped onion, red
- One cube cut tomato

DIRECTIONS

1. Add all the ingredients to a bowl and mix well.
2. Pour the dressing over the vegetable mixture and toss well to coat everything.
3. Serve and enjoy it.

NUTRITION: Calories: 93 cal Fat: 6 g Protein: 2 g Carbs: 9 g

8.5. Waldorf salad

Ready in: 20 minutes

Servings: 6

Difficulty: Easy

INGREDIENTS

- ½ cup raisins
- ½ cup mayonnaise
- 1 tsp lemon juice
- 1 tbsp sugar, white
- 1/8 tsp salt

- 1 cup celery stalk, sliced
- Three peeled and chopped apples
- ½ cup walnuts, chopped

DIRECTIONS

1. Combine salt, mayonnaise, lemon juice, and sugar in a mixing salad bowl.
2. Now add all the remaining ingredients and toss to coat.
3. Serve and enjoy it.

NUTRITION: Calories: 279 cal Fat: 21 g Protein: 2.3 g Carbs: 23.8 g

8.6. Chunky Tofu Guacamole

Ready in: 8 minutes

Servings: 12

Difficulty: Easy

INGREDIENTS

- ½ cup chopped red onion
- One avocado
- 7 oz salsa verde
- 12.3 oz tofu
- Two chopped garlic cloves
- ½ tsp salt
- One ¼ cups chopped tomato
- 2 tbsp lemon juice

DIRECTIONS

1. Remove the pulp from avocado and keep them aside.
2. Add salsa verde, tofu, garlic, lemon juice, salt, and avocado pulp in a blender.
3. Blend to obtain a smooth mixture.
4. Pour the mixture into the bowl.
5. Now add diced avocado, onion, and tomato into the blended mixture. Toss well.
6. Serve and enjoy it.

NUTRITION: Calories: 45 cal Fat: 2 g Protein: 2 g Carbs: 3 g

8.7. Creamy pasta salad

Ready in: 11 minutes

Servings: 6

Difficulty: Easy

INGREDIENTS

Salad

- ¼ cup green onions, sliced
- 8 oz salad pasta
- ½ cup chopped cucumber
- ½ cup black olives, sliced
- 1 cup broccoli florets
- ½ cup chopped red pepper

Dressing

- ½ tsp sugar
- ½ cup mayonnaise
- ½ tsp salt
- 2 tsp wine vinegar
- ½ tsp black pepper

DIRECTIONS

1. Using the instructions given over the package, cook pasta.
2. When pasta is almost done, stir in broccoli and let it cook with noodles for a minute.
3. Drain to remove excess water and wash them with cold water.
4. Combine sugar, mayonnaise, salt, vinegar, and black pepper in a container.

5. Transfer the mayonnaise mixture to noodle and broccoli bowl and toss well to coat everything.
6. Mix in pepper, onion, cucumber, and olives.
7. At this point, you can adjust the taste by adding pepper and salt.
8. Cover the bowl and place it in the refrigerator for few minutes.
9. Serve and enjoy it.

NUTRITION: Calories: 297 kcal Fat: 16 g Protein: 5 g Carbs: 31 g

8.8. Pear and Watercress Salad

Ready in: 15 minutes

Servings: 8

Difficulty: Easy

INGREDIENTS

Salad

- ½ cup goat cheese, crumbled
- 10 cups watercress
- ½ cup toasted walnuts
- One sliced peat
- 3 cups torn radicchio head
- One chopped fig, dried

Dressing

- ¼ cup olive oil
- 2 tbsp sherry vinegar
- 1 tsp maple syrup
- 1 tsp Dijon mustard
- ¼ tsp salt
- One minced shallot
- ¼ tsp pepper
- 1 tsp thyme, fresh

DIRECTIONS

1. Combine pepper, vinegar, maple syrup, salt, and Dijon mustard in a bowl and toss well.

2. Mix in thyme, oil, and shallot and whisk well.
3. The dressing is ready. Keep it aside until further use.
4. Add radicchio, walnuts, watercress, figs, and pear in a bowl. Toss.
5. Pour the dressing over the vegetable mixture and coat well.
6. Sprinkle cheese and serve.
7. Enjoy it.

NUTRITION: Calories: 163 cal Fat: 12 g Protein: 5 g Carbs: 10 g

Chapter 9: Vegetable Main Recipes

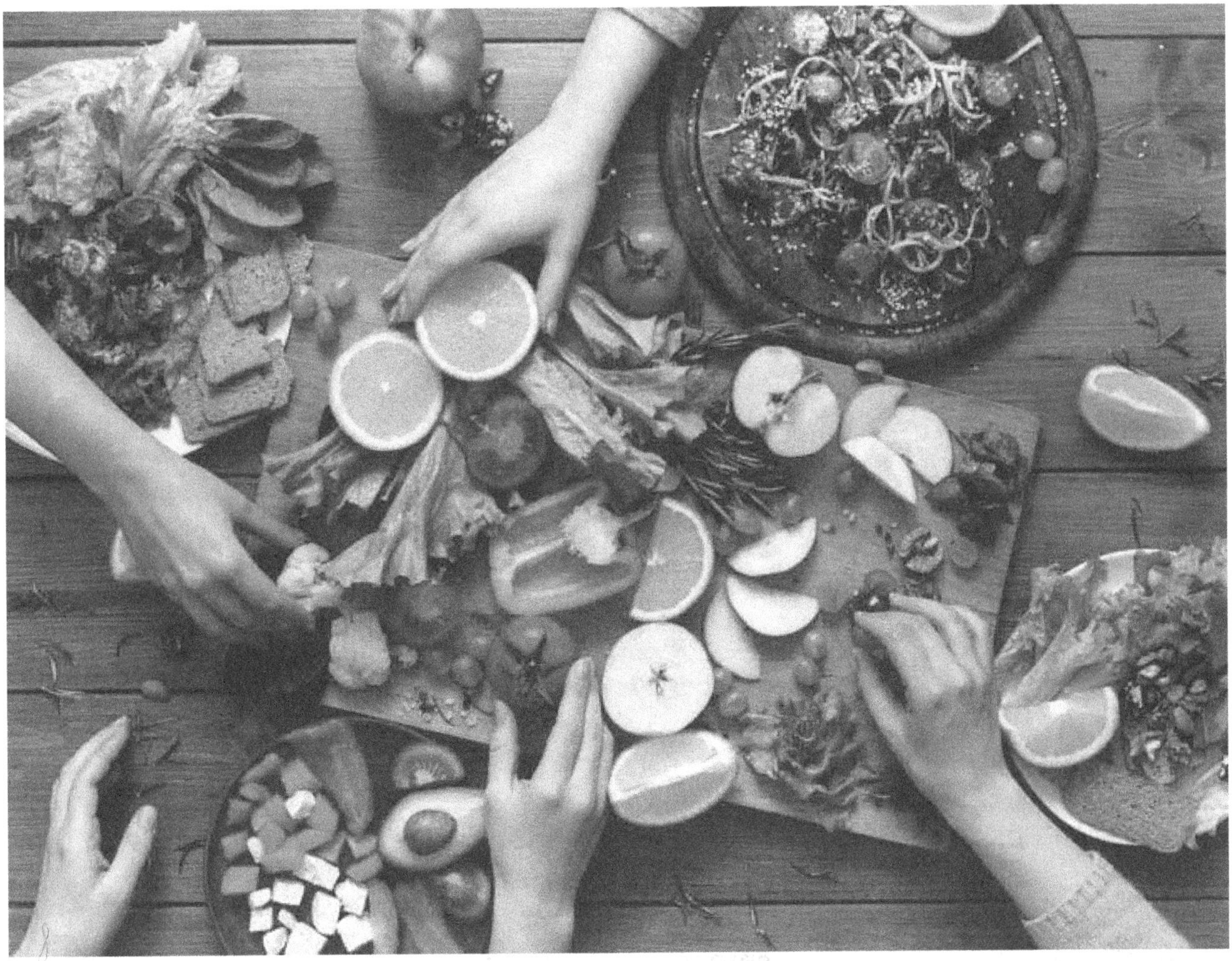

9.1. Vegetarian Pizza

Ready in: 45 minutes

Servings: 6

Difficulty: Medium

INGREDIENTS

- ½ cup sliced almonds
- Pizza dough
- ½ cup diced red onion
- 2 cups spinach
- 1 cup pizza sauce
- 3 cups grated mozzarella cheese
- ½ cup sliced bell pepper
- ½ cup sliced artichoke
- ½ cup Kalamata olives
- ½ cup cherry tomatoes
- Chopped basil for garnishing

DIRECTIONS

1. Divide the pizza dough into two portions or according to the size of the pan that you have for pizza.
2. Next, place pizza sauce and spread it over the dough.
3. Place spinach and cheese over the pizza dough.
4. Now spread the toppings over the cheese, such as bell pepper, olives,artichoke, almonds, tomatoes, and onions.
5. Bake the pizza in a preheated oven at 500 Fahrenheit for 12 minutes.
6. Place the pizza ins the serving plate and drizzle basil, cheese, and pepper flakes.

7. Serve and enjoy it.

NUTRITION: Calories: 440 cal Fat: 20.1 g Protein: 21.6 g Carbs: 44.9 g

9.2. Veggie Strata

Ready in: 120 minutes

Servings: 12

Difficulty: Difficult

INGREDIENTS

- 2 cups cheddar cheese
- 2 cups sliced Swiss chard
- Two chopped shallots
- ½ tsp kosher salt
- 4 tbsp butter
- Salt to taste
- 12 eggs
- 12 sliced bread
- Black pepper to taste
- 3 ½ cups milk
- ½ tsp grated nutmeg
- 2 tbsp Dijon mustard

DIRECTIONS

1. Melt the butter in a skillet over medium flame.
2. Cook shallots for few seconds.
3. Add salt and toss well.
4. Cook the shallots for five minutes with constant stirring.
5. Mix in chard and ¼ tsp of salt.
6. Cook for ten more minutes with frequent stirring.

7. Transfer the mixture to the plate and sprinkle black pepper and salt, and adjust the taste.
8. Keep it aside and let it cool. The green chard is ready.
9. Mix eggs, mustard, salt, milk, and nutmeg in a mixing bowl. Set aside.
10. Place bread pieces in the dish.
11. Add cooked green chard mixture over the bread pieces.
12. Spread cheese over the green and repeat the process for the second layer.
13. Now, pour the egg mixture over the bread pieces.
14. Cover the dish and place the dish in refrigerate for more than 4 hours.
15. Bake the mixture in a preheated oven at 350 Fahrenheit for 60 minutes.
16. Serve and enjoy it.

NUTRITION: Calories: 309 cal Fat: 17 g Protein: 19 g Carbs: 21 g

9.3. Veggie egg fried rice

Ready in: 15 minutes

Servings: 2

Difficulty: Easy

INGREDIENTS

- Soy sauce to taste
- 1 tbsp sunflower oil
- 1 ½ cup chopped pepper
- 1 tsp garlic puree
- 1 cup broccoli florets
- One egg
- 2 cups cooked rice

DIRECTIONS

1. Sauté garlic puree in heated oil over a high flame in a frying pan.
2. Stir in broccoli florets and peppers and cook for four minutes.
3. Mix in rice and fry for five more minutes.
4. Create a space in the middle of the rice and crack an egg in it.
5. Let it cook for two minutes.
6. Mix the egg in the rice and adjust the seasoning according to the taste.
7. Transfer the rice to the serving dish and drizzle some of the soy sauce.
8. Serve and enjoy it.

NUTRITION: Calories: 218 kcal Fat: 10 g Protein: 7 g Carbs: 26 g

9.4. **Coleslaw**

Ready in: 5 minutes

Servings: 2

Difficulty: Easy

INGREDIENTS

- ½ tsp black pepper
- 14 oz coleslaw mix
- 2 tbsp sugar
- ½ cup mayonnaise
- 1 ½ tbsp lemon juice
- ¼ tsp salt
- 1 tbsp vinegar

DIRECTIONS

1. Add all the ingredients to a large mixing bowl and toss everything well.
2. Mix in coleslaw and toss.
3. Place the bowl in refrigerate for three hours.
4. Serve and enjoy it.

NUTRITION: Calories: 240 cal Fat: 21 g Protein: 1 g Carbs: 12 g

9.5. Tabbouleh

Ready in: 35 minutes

Servings: 6

Difficulty: Medium

INGREDIENTS

- One minced garlic clove
- ½ cup bulgur
- 1 cup chopped tomato
- 1/3 cup sliced green onion
- 1 cup chopped cucumber
- 1 tsp salt
- 1/3 cup chopped mint
- 2 cups parsley
- 3 tbsp lime juice
- 1/3 cup olive oil

DIRECTIONS

1. Cook the bulgur as per the instructions written over the package. Transfer the cooked bulgur to a bowl and keep it aside.
2. Add cucumber, salt, and tomato to a bowl and mix well. Keep it aside until further use.
3. Mix bulgur, mint, chopped parsley, and onion in a bowl.
4. Drain off the excess liquid out of the tomato and cucumber mixture and mix them with bulgur mixture.
5. Combine oil, lemon juice, salt, and garlic and mix well.
6. Pour the lemon mixture over the bulgur mixture and toss well.

7. Adjust the taste by adding salt and lemon juice.

8. Let the salad rest for 20 minutes if possible for better taste.

9. Serve and enjoy it.

NUTRITION: Calories: 172 cal Fat: 13 g Protein: 3 g Carbs: 14 g

9.6. Couscous veggie patties

Ready in: 17 minutes

Servings: 8

Difficulty: Easy

INGREDIENTS

- 2 tbsp olive oil
- 2 cups cooked couscous
- Two chopped green onions
- Two eggs
- Two minced garlic clove
- ½ chopped red bell pepper
- 1 tsp ras el hanout
- 2 tbsp chopped parsley
- Salt to taste
- 2 tbsp flour

DIRECTIONS

1. Add all the ingredients to a large mixing bowl and mix well. The couscous mixture is ready to be cooked.
2. Heat olive oil in a skillet over medium flame.
3. Add a small portion of couscous mixture to the pan in the shape of couscous.
4. Let it cook for five minutes.
5. Press the batter with a spoon to give it a patty shape by keeping it in the skillet.
6. Now fry it for four minutes from both sides to get a golden color on either side.

7. Transfer the fried golden patties to a paper towel and dry them to remove excess oil.
8. Serve and enjoy it.

NUTRITION: Calories: 220 kcal Fat: 4.8 g Protein: 7.3 g Carbs: 36.2 g

9.7. Healthy spinach falafel

Ready in: 40 minutes

Servings: 4

Difficulty: Medium

INGREDIENTS

- 1 cup grated carrots
- 15 oz chickpeas
- ½ cup rolled oats
- Black pepper to taste
- 1/3 cup cilantro, fresh
- One chopped white onion
- Salt to taste
- 1 tbsp tahini
- 1 tsp cumin
- Four minced garlic cloves
- 1 cup spinach
- 1 tbsp lemon juice
- 2 tbsp sesame seeds

Tahini sauce

- Black pepper to taste
- ¼ cup tahini
- Water as required
- 2 tbsp lemon juice

DIRECTIONS

1. Combine all the ingredients in a blender, leaving sesame seeds, oats, and carrots on the shelf. Blend everything to get a smooth mixture.
2. Transfer the batter to a mixing bowl and add sesame seeds, carrots, and oats and toss well.
3. Make small balls out of the batter and place them onto the baking dish lined with parchment paper.
4. Bake the falafel in a preheated oven at 355 Fahrenheit for 35 minutes. Don't forget to change the falafel's sides at regular intervals to bake them from all the sides.
5. Mix all the items of tahini sauce in a bowl.
6. Spread the tahini sauce over the wraps and place baked falafel, and wrap it.
7. Serve and enjoy it.

NUTRITION: Calories: 247 kcal Fat: 10 g Protein: 8 g Carbs: 35 g

9.8. Ginger cranberry punch

Ready in: 15 minutes

Servings: 10

Difficulty: Easy

INGREDIENTS

- 12 oz cranberries
- ¾ cup water
- ¼ cup sliced ginger root
- ½ cup sugar
- ¼ cup lime juice
- 16 lime slices
- oz cranberry juice

DIRECTIONS

1. Add water in a saucepan and mix in gingerroot and sugar.
2. Bring it to boil over a high flame with occasional stirring to dissolve sugar in it.
3. Lower the flame to low and cover the pan. Let it simmer for five minutes.
4. Strain the solution and set it aside to cool it down.
5. Place the solution in the refrigerator to chill it.
6. Fill half of the serving cup with ginger syrup, then add lemon juice, cranberry juice, cranberries, and lemon slices.
7. Serve and enjoy it.

NUTRITION: Calories: 130 cal Fat: 0 g Protein: 0 g Carbs: 33 g

Chapter 10: Seafood Main Recipes

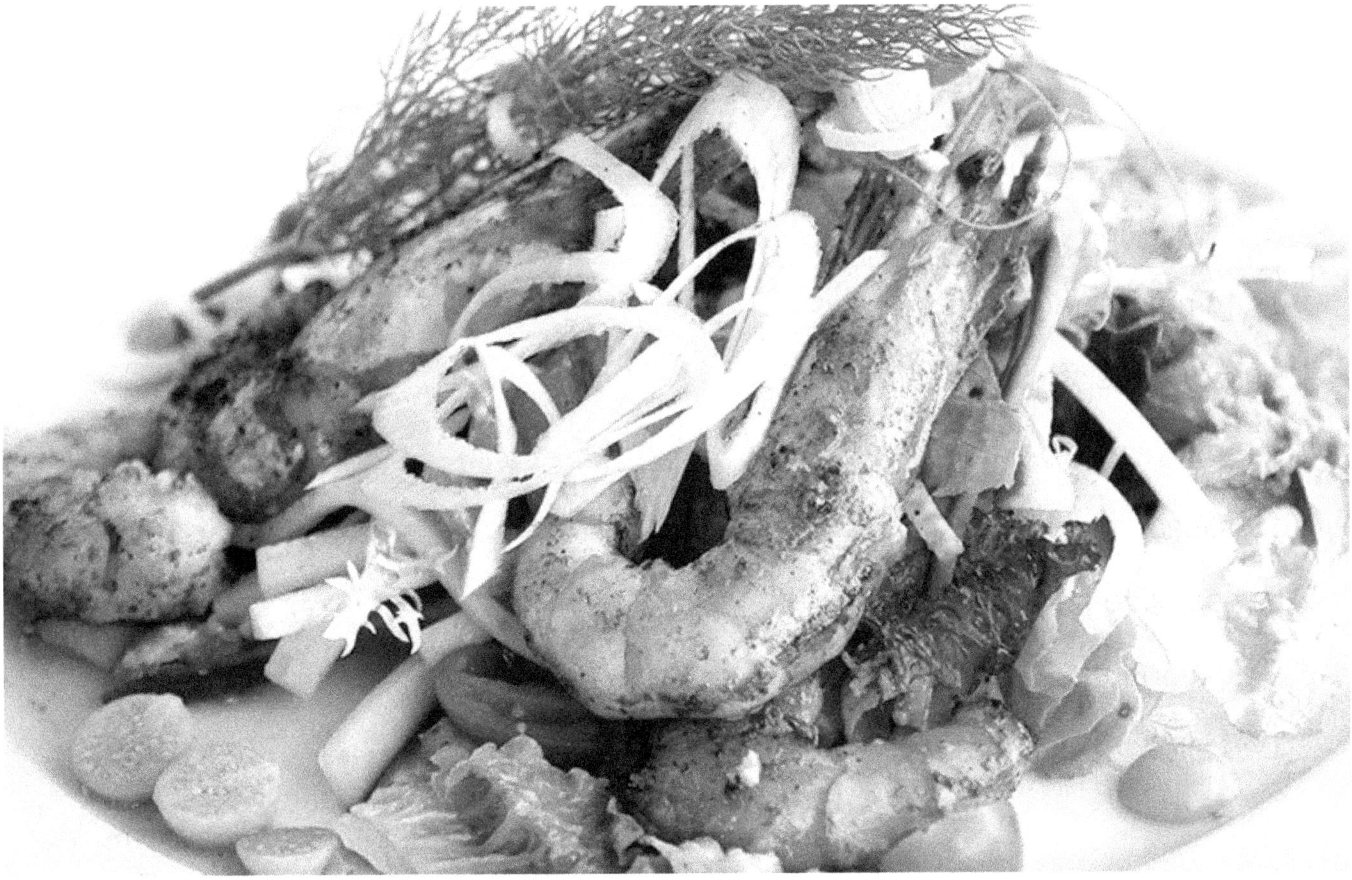

10.1. Baked fish with garlic and basil

Ready in: 26 minutes

Servings: 6

Difficulty: Easy

INGREDIENTS

- Two sliced shallots
- 2 lb fish
- 1 ½ tsp oregano, dried
- Salt to taste
- 2 tbsp lemon juice
- 1o minced garlic cloves
- Black pepper to taste
- 1 tsp sweet paprika
- 15 sliced basil leaves
- 6 tbsp olive oil
- 1 tsp coriander
- Two sliced bell pepper

DIRECTIONS

1. Rub fish with pepper and salt from both sides and set aside for a while.
2. Combine paprika, lemon juice, oregano, basil, coriander, olive oil, and garlic in a bowl and toss well.
3. Add fish in the bowl and toss well to coat fish with the marinade.
4. Place the bowl in the fridge for an hour.

5. Transfer the fish to a baking tray and place shallots and bell pepper around the fish.
6. Spread the marinade over the fish.
7. Bake in a preheated oven at 425 Fahrenheit for 15 minutes.
8. Remove the baked fish from the oven and place it in the serving dish.
9. Serve and enjoy it.

NUTRITION: Calories: 280 cal Fat: 16.2 g Protein: 28.8 g Carbs: 6 g

10.2. **Jambalaya**

Ready in: 55 minutes

Servings: 8

Difficulty: Medium

INGREDIENTS

- One bay leaf
- 3 tbsp olive oil
- 1 tsp thyme, dried
- 1 lb sliced andouille sausage
- Four minced garlic cloves
- Two chicken breast pieces, boneless
- 4 cups chicken broth
- Three diced bell pepper
- One chopped jalapeno pepper
- Two diced celery ribs
- One chopped white onion
- 14 oz crushed tomatoes
- 1 ½ cups white rice
- ¼ tsp cayenne pepper
- 1 cup sliced okra
- 1 lb raw shrimp
- Salt to taste
- Parsley for garnishing
- Black pepper to taste

- 2 tbsp Cajun seasoning
- Sliced green onions for garnishing

DIRECTIONS

1. Add olive oil to the pot and heat it over medium flame.
2. Stir in sausage and chicken and cook for eight minutes with constant stirring.
3. When chicken is fully done, transfer it to a plate and keep the plate aside for further use.
4. Again heat the olive oil in the same pot.
5. Sauté onion, bell pepper, garlic, jalapeno, and celery for seven minutes with occasional stirring.
6. When onion gets softened, stir in rice, bay leaf, thyme, tomatoes, cayenne, and Cajun seasoning and toss well.
7. Pour in chicken stock and let it simmer.
8. Lower the flame and cover the pot.
9. Simmer the solution for about 28 minutes with occasional stirring.
10. Now add okra and shrimp and toss.
11. Cook until shrimps turned pink.
12. Mix in sausage and chicken mixture and take away the bay leaf.
13. Sprinkle Cajun seasoning, pepper, and salt to adjust the taste.
14. Serve and enjoy it.
15. You can store it for four days by placing it in an airtight container.

NUTRITION: Calories: 576 kcal Fat: 22 g Protein: 43 g Carbs: 46 g

10.3. Crab cake stuffed shrimp

Ready in: 35 minutes

Servings: 12

Difficulty: Medium

INGREDIENTS

- 2 tbsp butter
- 2 tbsp butter
- ½ cup diced bell pepper (red and green)
- ½ cup diced onion
- One egg
- 24 jumbo shrimp
- 1 lb lump crabmeat
- 12 ritz crackers
- ½ cup panko crumbs
- Black pepper to taste
- 1 tsp bay seasoning
- ¼ tsp cayenne pepper
- ½ tsp lemon zest
- ½ cup mayonnaise
- Salt to taste

DIRECTIONS

1. Add bell pepper and onion in melted butter in a pan and cook for four minutes over medium flame.
2. Add crab, panko crumbs, black pepper, bay seasoning, mayo, crackers, egg, lemon zest, salt, and cayenne pepper. Toss well.

3. Place the deveined shrimps on the baking tray lined with parchment paper. Slightly press the shrimps.
4. Make balls out of crab mixture and place them over shrimps.
5. Spread melted butter over the crab mixture and shrimps.
6. Bake in a preheated oven at 350 Fahrenheit for 18 minutes.
7. Serve and enjoy it.

NUTRITION: Calories: 176 cal Fat: 2 g Protein: 4 g Carbs: 4 g

10.4. Tuscan Grilled Trout

Ready in: 20 minutes

Servings: 4

Difficulty: Easy

INGREDIENTS

- Eight trout fillets
- ¼ cup olive oil
- ½ tsp sage, dried
- One sliced garlic clove
- ½ tsp rosemary, dried
- ½ tsp salt
- 2 tbsp vinegar
- ¼ tsp black pepper

DIRECTIONS

1. Add olive oil to a pan and heat it over medium flame.
2. Stir in garlic, rosemary, and sage and cook for three minutes.
3. Remove the pan from flame and mix salt, vinegar, and pepper and toss well.
4. Now, place the trout fillets in the pan.
5. Add salt and vinegar mixture and toss well to coat trout.
6. Place the fish pieces over preheated grill keeping the skin side in a downwards direction.
7. Let it grill for three minutes.
8. After three minutes, check the fish's direction and cook from the other side for three minutes.
9. Transfer the grilled fish pieces to the plate.

10. Serve and enjoy it.

NUTRITION: Calories: 242 cal Fat: 12 g Protein: 31 g Carbs: 3.8 g

10.5. Seafood Casserole

Ready in: 60 minutes

Servings: 6

Difficulty: Medium

INGREDIENTS

- ¼ cup bread crumbs
- 6 oz rice
- 1 lb shrimp, cooked
- 1 lb crabmeat
- ½ tsp black pepper
- Two chopped celery ribs
- ½ cup chopped bell pepper, green
- Worcestershire sauce as required
- One chopped onion
- 4 oz mushroom
- 1 cup mayonnaise
- 2 oz chopped pimientos
- 1 cup milk

DIRECTIONS

1. Add water to a deep pan and bring it to a boil.
2. Stir in salt and rice and let the rice cook until they are done.
3. Drain the excess water and set it aside.
4. Mix bell pepper, pimientos, crab, onion, mushrooms, shrimp, and celery in a bowl and set aside.

5. Combine black pepper, mayo, Worcestershire, and milk in another bowl and whisk well.
6. Add the crab mixture to the mayo mixture and toss well.
7. In the last, add rice to the bowl and mix everything well.
8. Shift the mixture to a baking tray sprayed with oil.
9. Spread bread crumbs at the top.
10. Bake in a preheated oven at 375 Fahrenheit for 50 minutes.
11. Serve and enjoy it.

NUTRITION: Calories: 585 cal Fat: 34 g Protein: 37 g Carbs: 31 g

10.6. Baked Lemon Garlic Halibut

Ready in: 25 minutes

Servings: 4

Difficulty: Easy

INGREDIENTS

- 2 tbsp chopped parsley
- 3 tbsp olive oil
- 1 tsp smoked paprika
- 1/3 cup lemon juice
- One chopped tomato
- ½ tsp pepper flakes
- ½ tsp black pepper
- Six smashed garlic cloves
- 1 tsp salt
- 1 lb halibut fillet
- 1 tsp dill, dried

DIRECTIONS

1. Whisk parsley, olive oil, lemon juice, garlic, salt, black pepper, pepper flakes, paprika, and dill in a bowl.
2. Add halibut fillet in a bowl and toss well to coat fillets with the marinade.
3. Cover the bowl and place it in the fridge for three hours to marinate.
4. Transfer the fillets to a baking tray and bake in a preheated oven at 350 Fahrenheit for 22 minutes.
5. Serve with tomatoes and parsley and enjoy it.

NUTRITION: Calories: 216 kcal Fat: 12 g Protein: 21 g Carbs: 4 g

10.7. Salmon Burger

Ready in: 20 minutes

Servings: 4

Difficulty: Easy

INGREDIENTS

- 2 tbsp Lemon wedges
- 1 ½ lb salmon, boneless
- 2 tbsp butter
- Two shallots
- 2 tsp Dijon mustard
- ½ cup bread crumbs
- Salt to taste
- 1 tbsp capers
- Pepper to taste
- Tabasco sauce as required

DIRECTIONS

1. Add chopped salmon and mustard in a blender and blend to get a mixture.
2. Now add the shallots and blend again.
3. Transfer the blended mixture to a bowl and stir in bread crumbs, salt, capers, and pepper.
4. Mix everything using hands.
5. Make flat patties out of the batter of the required size.
6. Melt butter in a skillet over medium flame.
7. Add patties and cook for five minutes from each side.

8. Serve and enjoy it.

NUTRITION: Calories: 461 cal Fat: 20 g Protein: 37 g Carbs: 32 g

10.8. Fish Chowder

Ready in: 55 minutes

Servings: 6

Difficulty: Medium

INGREDIENTS

- 2 tbsp chopped parsley
- One olive oil
- 2 cups chopped yellow onion
- 1 tbsp thyme, fresh
- 1 tsp butter
- 1 ½ tsp salt
- ½ cup white wine, dried
- 2 cups clam juice
- Three cubes cut potatoes
- 1 ½ cup heavy cream
- One bay leaf
- 1 tsp bay seasoning
- ¼ tsp black pepper
- 1 ½ lb cod

DIRECTIONS

1. Sauté onions in heated oil in a pot over medium flame for five minutes.
2. Pour in the wine and mix well.
3. Increase the flame and cook to reduce the wine content to half.

4. Stir in clam juice, pepper, bay leaf, potatoes, salt, bay spice, and thyme. Mix well.
5. Reduce the flame and let it simmer.
6. Cover the pot and cook for 15 minutes.
7. Add cream to another pot and let it simmer over medium flame.
8. Transfer the steamed cream to the potato mixture and stir in fish.
9. Cook the mixture over low flame for 12 minutes.
10. Stir in parsley and remove the pot from the flame.
11. Let it rest for half an hour.
12. Serve and enjoy it.

NUTRITION: Calories: 386 cal Fat: 13.6 g Protein: 31.9 g Carbs: 33.8 g

Chapter 11: Poultry and Meat Main Recipes

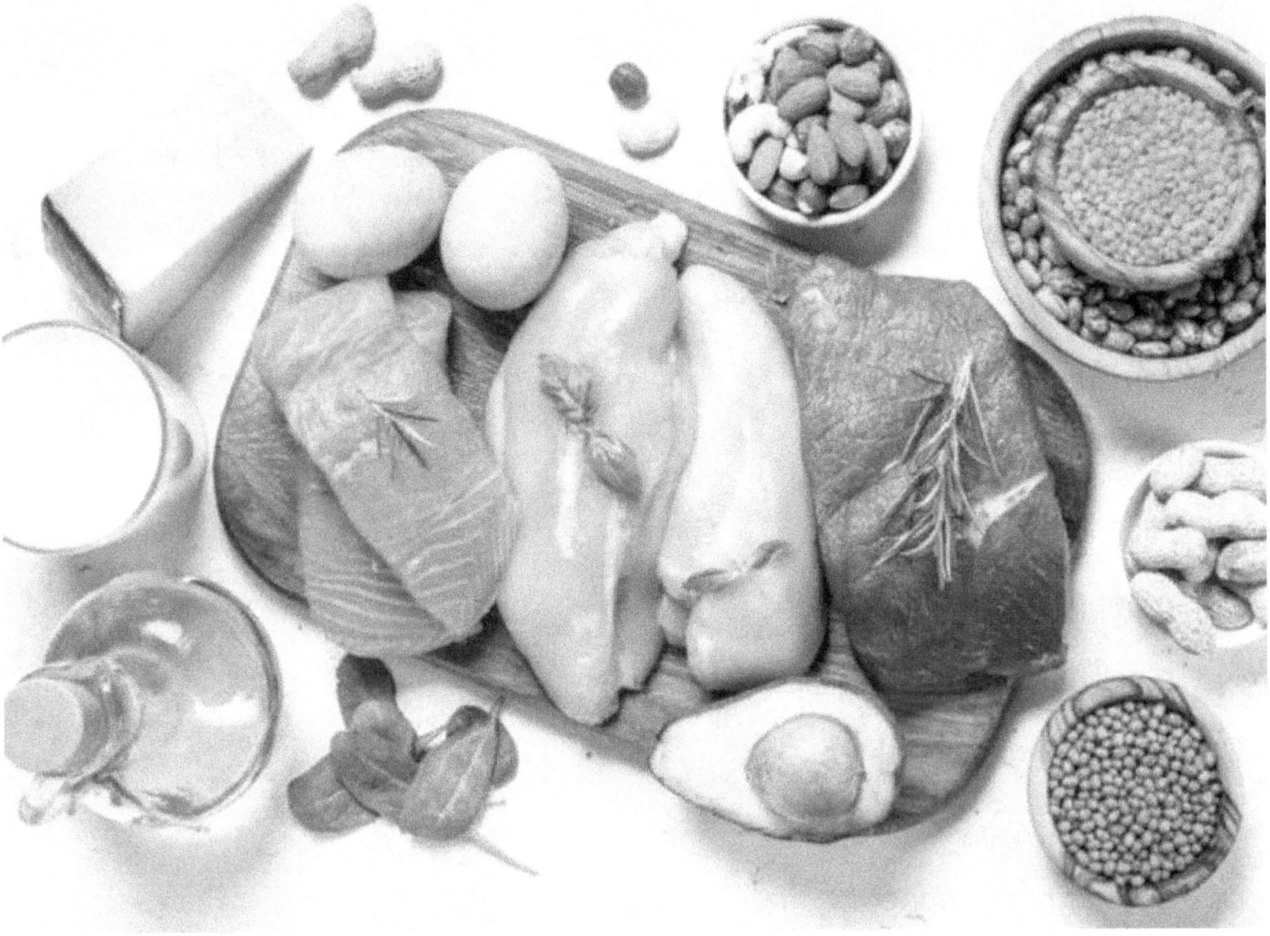

11.1. Asian Steak Wraps

Ready in: 30 minutes

Servings: 4

Difficulty: Medium

INGREDIENTS

- 2 tsp toasted sesame seeds
- ¼ cup lime juice
- 1 tbsp soy sauce
- 3 tbsp honey
- 2 tsp sesame oil
- One diced sweet red pepper
- 1 ½ tsp chopped cilantro
- 2 tsp smashed ginger root
- 1 lb sliced beef steak
- ¼ tsp pepper
- ¼ tsp salt
- One sliced onion
- Four tortillas
- One sliced green pepper
- 2 oz cream cheese

DIRECTIONS

1. Combine sesame seeds, lime juice, soy sauce, honey, ginger root, cilantro, salt, and pepper in a bowl and whisk.
2. Divide the marinade into two parts, such as 2/3 and 1/3.

3. Add beef in 1/3 of the marinade and toss.
4. Place the beef coated marinade bowl in the fridge.
5. Cover the second 2/3 marinade and set aside.
6. Fry beef in heated oil and cook until turning brown and all the pink color diminishes.
7. Transfer the fried beef pieces to the plate.
8. Sauté bell pepper and onions in the same pan.
9. Pour in the 2/3 part of the marinade and cook for three minutes.
10. Add fried beef pieces into the pan and cook over medium flame.
11. Spread cream cheese over the tortillas and place the beef mixture over it.
12. Drizzle sesame seeds and fold the tortillas.
13. Serve and enjoy it.

NUTRITION: Calories: 402 cal Fat: 14 g Protein: 29 g Carbs: 41 g

11.2. **Roast Beef**

Ready in: 190 minutes

Servings: 8

Difficulty: Difficult

INGREDIENTS

- 1 tsp black pepper
- 4 lb round roast
- Three minced garlic cloves
- ¼ cup olive oil
- 1 tbsp diced rosemary
- 2 tsp salt
- 1 tbsp chopped thyme

DIRECTIONS

1. Whisk rosemary, oil, salt, garlic, black pepper, and thyme in a bowl.
2. Add the roast pieces to the rosemary mixture and coat the pieces well.
3. Put the pieces in a roasting pan and let them roast for 17 minutes in a preheated oven at 420 Fahrenheit.
4. After 17 minutes, decrease the oven temperature to 325 degrees Fahrenheit and let it roast for 105 minutes.
5. Serve and enjoy it with your favorite dipping sauce.

NUTRITION: Calories: 564 cal Fat: 35 g Protein: 52.8 g Carbs: 9.8 g

11.3. Lemon Herb Turkey Breast

Ready in: 140 minutes

Servings: 10

Difficulty: Difficult

INGREDIENTS

- One lemon
- 6 lb turkey breast
- 2 tsp mustard, dried
- 1 tsp chopped thyme leaves
- 1 tbsp minced garlic
- 1 tbsp chopped rosemary leaves
- 2 tbsp lemon juice
- 1 tbsp chopped sage leaves
- 1 tbsp salt
- 2 tbsp olive oil
- ½ tbsp black pepper
- 1 cup chicken stock

DIRECTIONS

1. Spray the baking rack with oil and set it aside.
2. Place breast pieces on the rack with the skin side facing upwards.
3. Whisk mustard, olive oil, garlic, salt, lemon juice, mustard, black pepper, and herbs in a bowl.
4. Rub the marinade over the breast pieces and spread the remaining mixture over the pieces.
5. Add the chicken stock to the roasting pan and add lemon pieces to it.
6. Bake the breast pieces in a preheated oven at 325 Fahrenheit for two hours.
7. Serve and enjoy it.

NUTRITION: Calories: 440 kcal Fat: 20 g Protein: 59 g Carbs: 1 g

11.4. Chicken satay

Ready in: 60 minutes

Servings: 4

Difficulty: Difficult

INGREDIENTS

- Olive oil as required
- 2 lb chicken pieces, boneless
- One sliced onion
- One sliced cucumber

Marination

- 2 tbsp honey
- 3 tbsp oil
- 1 tsp coriander powder
- Two garlic cloves
- 1 tsp chili powder
- Two lemongrass stalks
- ½ tsp salt
- Six chopped pearly onions
- 2 tsp turmeric powder

DIRECTIONS

1. Slice the chicken pieces in cube shape and place them in a bowl. Keep the bowl aside for a while.

2. Add honey, oil, chili powder, lemongrass, turmeric powder, salt, garlic, onion, and coriander powder in a blender and blend to get a smooth mixture. You can use a few tbsp of water if you need the feel for it.
3. Transfer the mixture to a bowl. The marinade is ready.
4. Add chicken cubes into the marinade and toss well to coat the chicken cubes with marinade.
5. Place the bowl in the fridge for overnight to get the best results.
6. Thread the chicken pieces over the skewers.
7. Preheat the grill.
8. Place the skewers on the grill and cook for five minutes from each side.
9. Keep brushing the chicken cubes with oil during cooking.
10. When the chicken is fully done, transfer the cubes to the plate.
11. Serve and enjoy it.

NUTRITION: Calories: 263 cal Fat: 14 g Protein: 31 g Carbs: 13 g

11.5. Cilantro lime chicken drumsticks

Ready in: 90 minutes

Servings: 4

Difficulty: Difficult

INGREDIENTS

- Six chicken drumsticks
- 2 tbsp oil
- ½ tsp cumin
- ½ cup chopped cilantro
- Four minced garlic cloves
- ½ tsp salt
- Two limes
- Cracker pepper to taste

DIRECTIONS

1. Add pepper, cumin, oil, salt, and garlic in a mixing bowl.
2. Remove the lime zest using a grater and add in the garlic mixture.
3. Stir in lime juice and toss well.
4. Chop the cilantro and add them to a container and mix well. The marinade is ready to be used.
5. Mix chicken drumsticks in the container and toss to coat the chicken with the marinade.
6. Cover the bowl and place it in the fridge for one hour or longer to get a better taste.
7. Arrange the chicken drumsticks in a baking tray.
8. Pour the marinade over the chicken pieces in a baking tray.

9. Bake in a preheated oven at 400 Fahrenheit for 44 minutes.
10. Brush the pieces with oil during baking twice.
11. For the last five minutes, turn on the broiler mode and broil to get good results.
12. Sprinkle cilantro leaves and place line slices over the baked chicken.
13. Serve and enjoy it.

NUTRITION: Calories: 528.6 kcal Fat: 33.57 g Protein: 48.6 g Carbs: 7.13 g

11.6. **BBQ Beef Cups**

Ready in: 40 minutes

Servings: 6

Difficulty: Medium

INGREDIENTS

- 1/3 cup grated cheddar cheese
- ¾ lb ground beef
- 1 tbsp dried onion
- ½ cup BBQ sauce
- 12 oz biscuit dough

DIRECTIONS

1. Add beef in a skillet and cook over medium flame until beef is done.
2. Remove the extra fat releases during the cooking of beef.
3. Add onion and BBQ sauce and mix well.
4. Reduce the flame and bring it to simmer for 10 minutes.
5. Break the biscuits and add them to muffin cups and press them slightly.
6. Add meat mixture at the top of the crumbled biscuits.
7. Bake for 15 minutes in a preheated oven at 350 Fahrenheit.
8. After 15 minutes, add cheese and bake again for five minutes to melt the cheese.
9. Remove the pan from the oven and let it rest for few minutes.
10. Serve and enjoy it.

NUTRITION: Calories: 353 cal Fat: 17.2 g Protein: 16.5 g Carbs: 32.4 g

11.7. Jalapeno Popper Chicken

Ready in: 45 minutes

Servings: 6

Difficulty: Medium

INGREDIENTS

- 1 cup grated cheddar cheese
- 2 lb chicken breast pieces, boneless
- Two diced jalapeno pepper
- Salt to taste
- 2 tbsp milk
- Pepper to taste
- ½ tsp garlic powder
- 8 oz cream cheese
- ½ cup cooked bacon

DIRECTIONS

1. Place the chicken pieces in a baking tray sprayed with oil in one layer.
2. Sprinkle pepper and salt over the chicken pieces.
3. Combine cream cheese, garlic powder, and milk in a mixing bowl.
4. You can slightly heat the mixture to make it easy for yourself to whisk them.
5. Pour the mixture over the chicken pieces in a baking tray.
6. Spread cheese, jalapeno, and bacon pieces over the top of the chicken placed in a baking tray.
7. Cover the tray with foil.
8. Bake in a preheated oven at 350 Fahrenheit for 33 minutes until the chicken is tenderized completely.

9. Take away the foil and bake to melt the cheese completely for seven more minutes.
10. Serve and enjoy it.

NUTRITION: Calories: 349 cal Fat: 26 g Protein: 28 g Carbs: 1 g

11.8. **Pan Sausage**

Ready in: 25 minutes

Servings: 6

Difficulty: Easy

INGREDIENTS

- 2 lb pork
- 2 tsp sage, dried
- 1/8 tsp pepper flakes
- 2 tsp salt
- 1 tbsp brown sugar
- 1 tsp black pepper
- ¼ tsp ground clove
- ¼ tsp marjoram, dried

DIRECTIONS

1. Whisk sage, marjoram, cloves, salt, red pepper, black pepper, and sugar in a bowl.
2. Add the pork pieces and mix everything well using your hands.
3. Make required sized patties out of the batter.
4. Heat oil in a skillet over medium flame.
5. Fry patties in the heated oil for five minutes from both sides.
6. When patties turned brown from both sides, transfer them into the serving dish.
7. Serve and enjoy it.

NUTRITION: Calories: 409 cal Fat: 32.2 g Protein: 25.6 g Carbs: 2.7 g

Chapter 12: Desserts Recipes

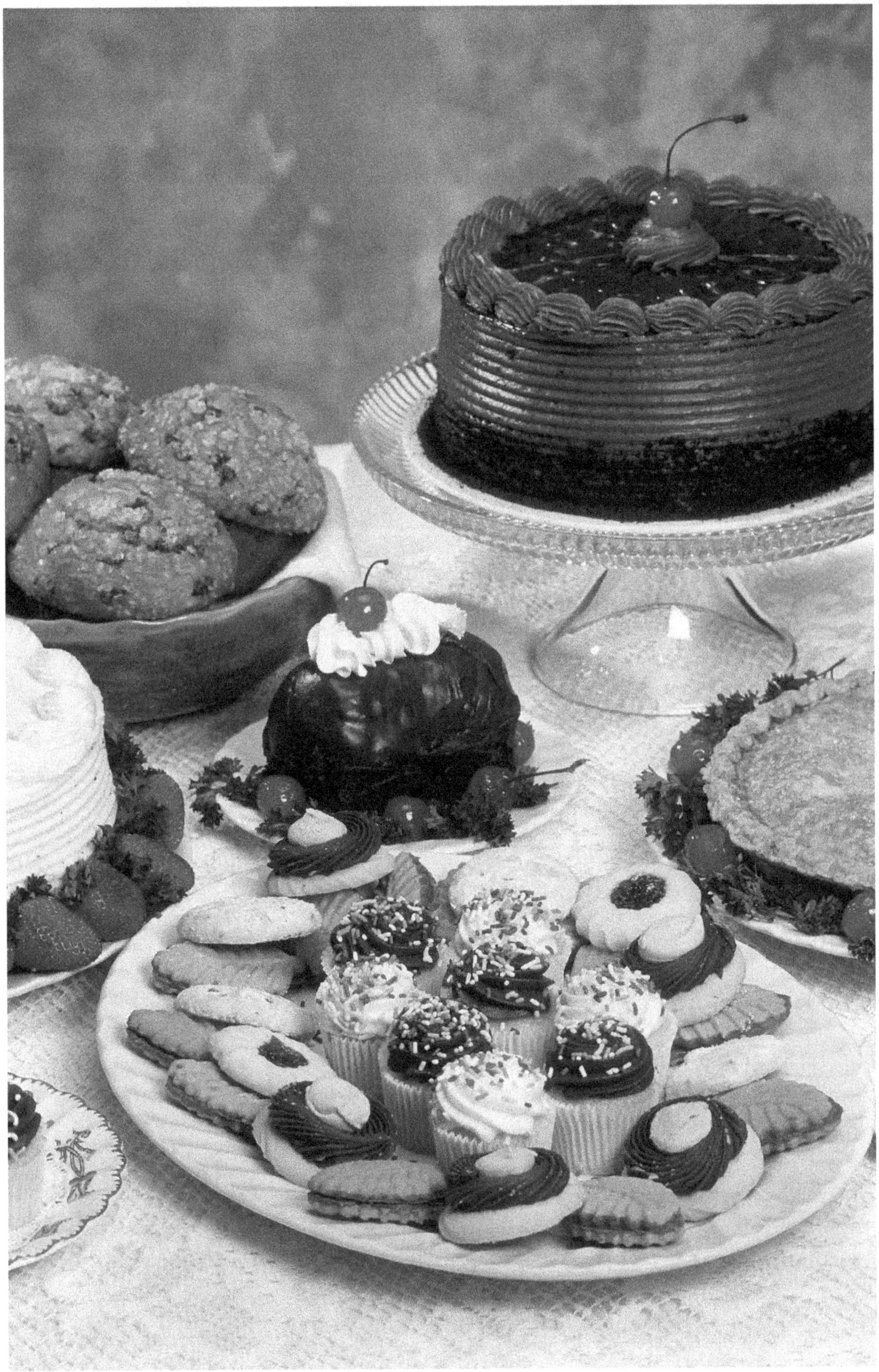

12.1. Lemon thins

Ready in: 24 minutes

Servings: 24 cookies

Difficulty: Easy

INGREDIENTS

- 1 cup all-purpose flour
- 6 oz butter
- 2 tbsp lemon zest, grated
- ¼ tsp baking soda
- 1 ½ cups sugar
- 1 tbsp lemon juice
- One egg
- 1 tsp lemon extract
- ¼ tsp salt

DIRECTIONS

1. Mix lemon zest, lemon juice, butter, and lemon extract, including sugar and egg, and mix them well.
2. After it, mix salt, flour, and baking soda in the mixture.
3. Spread on the sheet using a scoop.
4. Cook then for 9 to 10 minutes until brown color appears on edges.
5. After cooling, serve them.

NUTRITION: Calories: 49 cal Fat: 2 g Protein: 0 g Carbs: 7 g

12.2. Classic Peanut Butter Cookies

Ready in: 25 minutes

Servings: 24 cookies

Difficulty: Easy

INGREDIENTS

- 1 ½ tsp baking soda
- 1 cup butter
- 1 cup sugar, white
- ½ tsp salt
- 1 cup peanut butter
- 1 cup brown sugar
- 2 ½ cups all-purpose flour
- Two eggs
- 1 tsp baking powder

DIRECTIONS

1. Whisk egg, cream butter, sugar, and peanut butter in a bowl. Set aside for a while.
2. Combine baking soda, flour, and baking powder in another bowl and mix well.
3. Add the dry ingredient mixture in butter mixture and mix to get a smooth mixture.
4. Place the bowl in the fridge for one hour.
5. Make small balls out of the dough and place them in a baking tray.
6. Press the balls using a spoon to form a sheet. Make a pattern of your choice using a fork.
7. Bake in a preheated oven at 375 Fahrenheit for 10 minutes.

8. Place the flat rounded dough in a baking tray.
9. Serve and enjoy it.

NUTRITION: Calories: 252 cal Fat: 13.6 g Protein: 4.5 g Carbs: 29.7 g

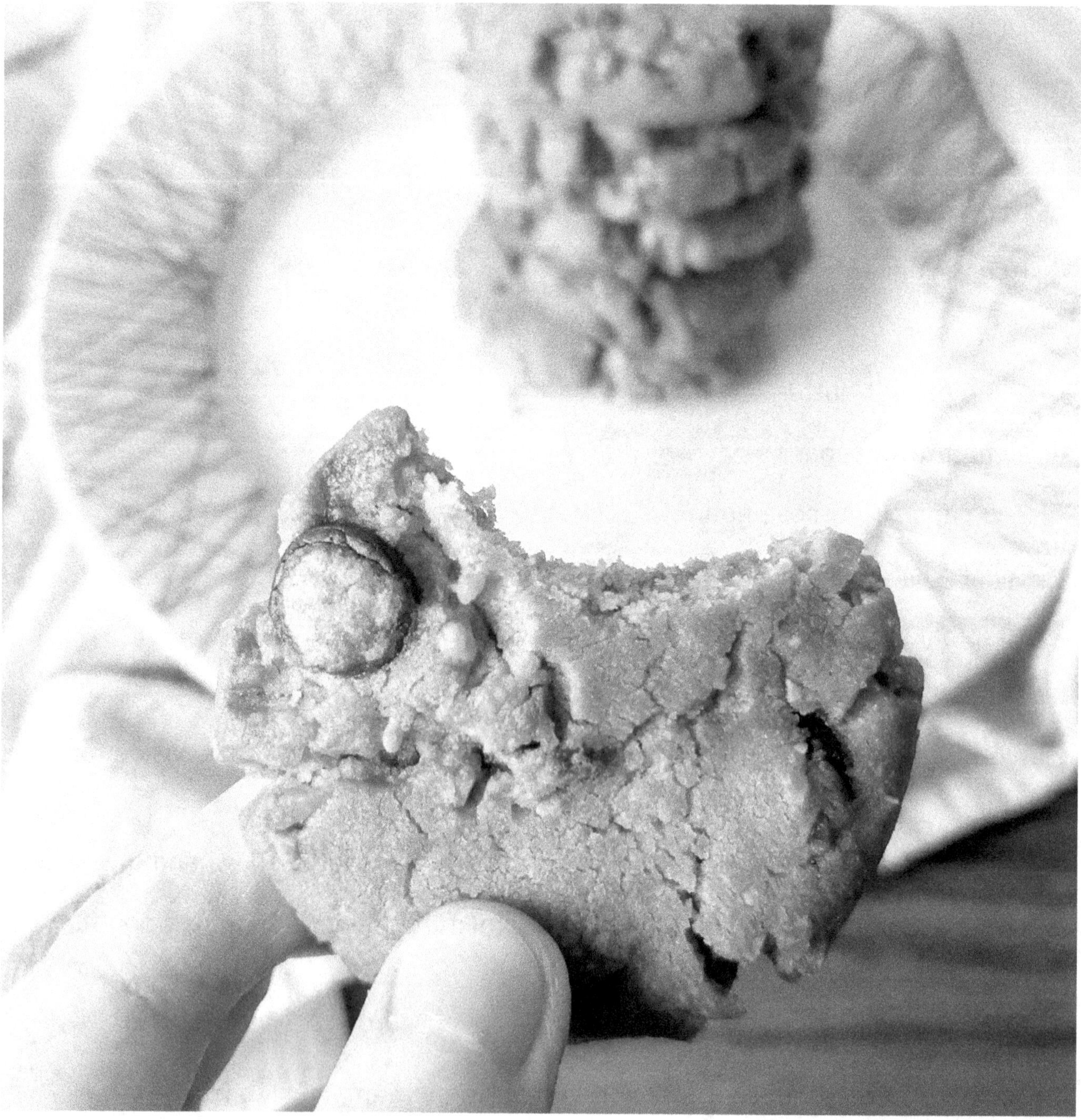

12.3. Blueberry Cheesecake

Ready in: 100 minutes

Servings: 12

Difficulty: Medium

INGREDIENTS

Cheesecake base

- 8 tbsp butter
- 7 oz plain biscuits

Cheesecake filling

- 8 oz blueberries
- 1 lb cream cheese
- 1 tsp vanilla extract
- 2 tbsp flour
- ½ cup sour cream
- 2 tbsp lemon zest
- 1 ½ cups sugar, caster
- Three eggs

Blueberry topping

- 2 tbsp water
- 13 oz blueberries
- 1 ½ tsp cornstarch
- ½ cup white sugar
- 2 tbsp lemon juice
- ½ tsp vanilla extract

DIRECTIONS

1. Prepare the base with baking paper having oil or butter speared.
2. In a mixer, mix butter and biscuits and put them in a prepared base.
3. For the filling, blend the cheese for 1/3 of a minute. Combine it with flour and blend for five seconds after mixing it with sugar, vanilla, lemon zest, and sour cream.
4. Then mix them with egg one by one, blend each time for five seconds, and finally mix in blueberries.
5. Cook it for 1hour and a minute.

Blueberry sauce for cheesecake

1. On low to medium flame, mix lemon juice, blueberries, sugar, and vanilla for six to seven minutes.
2. Add water and cornflour and mix it well till it got thicken.
3. Combine all blueberries and cool them.
4. Pour it in the cheesecake fully,
5. Slice it and serve and enjoy!

NUTRITION: Calories: 489 cal Fat: 28 g Protein: 5 g Carbs: 55 g

12.4. Clementine chocolate lava cake

Ready in: 20 minutes

Servings: 4

Difficulty: Easy

INGREDIENTS

- ½ cup olive oil
- 4 oz chocolate bar
- 2 cups sugar
- Two eggs
- 1/8 tsp salt
- 4 tbsp clementine zest
- 1 tsp vanilla
- Cocoa powder to garnish

DIRECTIONS

1. Oil the pan and heat it on two hundred C0.
2. Mix the olive oil, salt, egg, clementine zest, vanilla, and sugar, and mix it with melted chocolate.
3. Cook it for 9 to 11 minutes.
4. Spread the cocoa powder and clementine.
5. Serve and enjoy

NUTRITION: Calories: 624 kcal Fat: 33 g Protein: 6 g Carbs: 71 g

12.5. Carrot cake

Ready in: 55 minutes

Servings: 12

Difficulty: Medium

INGREDIENTS

- 2 cups grated carrots
- 2 cups chopped pecans
- ½ cup granulated sugar
- 1 ½ cup brown sugar
- ¼ tsp nutmeg
- 1 cup canola oil
- ¾ cup applesauce
- Four eggs
- ¼ tsp cloves
- 2 tsp baking powder
- 1 tsp vanilla extract
- ½ tsp salt
- 2 ½ cups all-purpose flour
- 1 tsp baking soda
- 1 tsp ginger
- 1 ½ tsp cinnamon

Cream cheese frosting

- ¼ tsp salt
- 1 ½ tsp vanilla extract

- 16 oz cream cheese
- 4 ½ cup sugar
- ½ cup butter
- 1 tbsp milk

DIRECTIONS

1. Sprinkled the pecans over a baking sheet and cooked it for 10 minutes at 145 to 150 degrees.
2. Mix the vanilla, brown sugar, applesauce, oil, eggs, and granulated sugar; on another side, combine cloves, cinnamon, baking powder, salt, ginger, nutmeg, flour, and baking soda. Combine wet and dry components, fold these ingredients in carrots and pecans. In cake pans, cook it for 25 to 30 minutes.
3. For the frosting, mix the cream, butter, and cheese with a blender for 120 seconds. Mix sugar, salt, cream, and vanilla extract, also beat for half a minute.
4. To assemble and frost, cut the cake layers using a knife, cover the top layer of cake with frosting evenly, and top up the second layer with more frosting and then over the third layer of the cake.
5. Spread the frosting on the sides and also on top of it. Decorate it with pecans. Cool, serve, and enjoy it.

NUTRITION: Calories: 535 cal Fat: 33.4 g Protein: 5.6 g Carbs: 56.4 g

12.6. Sunburst Lemon Bars

Ready in: 120 minutes

Servings: 36

Difficulty: Difficult

INGREDIENTS

Base

- ½ cup sugar
- 2 cups all-purpose flour
- 1 cup butter

Filling

- ¼ cup lemon juice
- Four eggs
- ¼ cup all-purpose flour
- 2 cups sugar, granulated
- 1 tsp baking powder

Glaze

- 3 tbsp lemon juice
- 1 cup sugar

DIRECTIONS

1. In a pan, mix main components with blender and cook it for half an hour.
2. In another pan, mix the egg with all other components and finally add lemon juice and blend it.
3. Add filling on cooked base. After adding, cook it for half an hour and cool it down.
4. Add lemon juice in sugar, stir it, and pour it on cooled bars.

NUTRITION: Calories: 150 cal Fat: 6 g Protein: 2 g Carbs: 22 g

12.7. Baked Egg Custard

Ready in: 45 minutes

Servings: 4

Difficulty: Medium

INGREDIENTS

- ½ cup sugar
- Three eggs
- 1 tsp vanilla extract
- One egg yolk
- 2 cups cream
- Grated nutmeg for garnishing

DIRECTIONS

1. Blend vanilla extract, egg, and yolk of eggs. Mix the sugar with cream in a pan on low flame and mix it with eggs. Stand over a pan filled with hot water Spread nutmeg on the top. Cook it for half an hour
2. Then serve it and enjoy it with chilled, steamed fruits.

NUTRITION: Calories: 219 kcal Fat: 47 g Protein: 9 g Carbs: 19 g

12.8. Pomegranate Smoothie

Ready in: 5 minutes

Servings: 2

Difficulty: Easy

INGREDIENTS

- 1 cup pomegranate juice
- 1 cup diced pears

- ¼ cup pomegranate arils
- One banana
- 2 tbsp smashed ginger
- 2 cups strawberries, frozen
- 1 cup ice cubes

DIRECTIONS

1. Combine all the ingredients in a bowl and toss well.
2. Transfer the mixture to a food processor and blend to get a smooth mixture.

COOKING CONVERSION CHART

Measurement

CUP	ONCES	MILLILITERS	TABLESPOONS
8 cup	64 oz	1895 ml	128
6 cup	48 oz	1420 ml	96
5 cup	40 oz	1180 ml	80
4 cup	32 oz	960 ml	64
2 cup	16 oz	480 ml	32
1 cup	8 oz	240 ml	16
3/4 cup	6 oz	177 ml	12
2/3 cup	5 oz	158 ml	11
1/2 cup	4 oz	118 ml	8
3/8 cup	3 oz	90 ml	6
1/3 cup	2.5 oz	79 ml	5.5
1/4 cup	2 oz	59 ml	4
1/8 cup	1 oz	30 ml	3
1/16 cup	1/2 oz	15 ml	1

Temperature

FAHRENHEIT	CELSIUS
100 °F	37 °C
150 °F	65 °C
200 °F	93 °C
250 °F	121 °C
300 °F	150 °C
325 °F	160 °C
350 °F	180 °C
375 °F	190 °C
400 °F	200 °C
425 °F	220 °C
450 °F	230 °C
500 °F	260 °C
525 °F	274 °C
550 °F	288 °C

Weight

IMPERIAL	METRIC
1/2 oz	15 g
1 oz	29 g
2 oz	57 g
3 oz	85 g
4 oz	113 g
5 oz	141 g
6 oz	170 g
8 oz	227 g
10 oz	283 g
12 oz	340 g
13 oz	369 g
14 oz	397 g
15 oz	425 g
1 lb	453 g

3. Pour the thick creamy juice into serving glasses.
4. Serve and enjoy it.

NUTRITION: Calories: 218 cal Fat: 0.2 g Protein: 2 g Carbs: 54 g

Conclusion

Due to insignificant symptoms, kidney disease is difficult to diagnose at the initial stages. People who are already suffering from diabetes or high blood pressure are more prone to catching this disease. It is important to pinpoint this disease at the initial level to avoid further complications. A kidney transplant is the best option to escape this failure, but it needs a kidney donor. Meanwhile, dialysis is another option that needs to be performed repeatedly, making it an expensive and temporary fix. Suppose the patient's kidney is still managing to work to some extent. In that case, it is advised to follow the patient's physician's renal diet to avoid further worsening kidney condition. A renal diet will help control kidney failure, but it will also control cholesterol levels, blood pressure, blood sugar, and other problems. In a renal diet, the main focus is to cut back salt, maintain the balance of phosphorous, keep blood sugar at an optimum degree and keep phosphate level at its best.

Along with that, it helps reduce protein intake excess of which can put the kidney in trouble. It is important to note that every disease has its cure; the only thing required from the patient is to remain determined and religiously follow physician instructions. Renal diet can impart new taste to patient's life with its diverse kind of meals and their recipes

CPSIA information can be obtained
at www.ICGtesting.com
Printed in the USA
LVHW061017090122
707896LV00022B/172